Advance praise for *Better Medicine: Reforming Canadian Health Care*

"*Better Medicine* is well written, interesting, and thought-provoking. While many think of the current health care system as cast in stone, and some prophesy dire consequences should we attempt to change it, this book makes a cogent case for reform. The contributors describe both the economic flaws and the human costs of the status quo, and provide timely ideas for improvement."

— WILLIAM ROBSON

Vice President and Director of Research,
C.D. Howe Institute

"There is no question that Canadians will face some tough choices in deciding how to organize and pay for health care in the future. If the status quo remains, there will be increasing shortages and very, very long waits for urgent and necessary health care. This book exhorts Canadians to look outside the ideologically based constraints imposed by one side of the political spectrum. Even if we might not choose to adopt any of the ideas presented in *Better Medicine*, we owe it to ourselves to at least give them a serious look."

— DR. ALLAN S. DETSKY

Professor of Medicine and Health Policy Management and Evaluation,
University of Toronto

About the Editor

Dr. David Gratzer is a physician and writer. He is the author of *Code Blue* (ECW Press, 1999), which was awarded the Donner Prize for the best Canadian public policy book in 2000. He is often quoted on health matters both in Canada and the United States and is frequently invited to speak on health reform. He contributes regularly to the *National Post* and *The Medical Post*. He has written for more than a dozen newspapers and magazines, including *The Globe and Mail*, *The Ottawa Citizen*, and *Time*.

Dr. Gratzer lives in Toronto.

BETTER MEDICINE

BETTER MEDICINE

Reforming Canadian Health Care

Edited by Dr. David Gratzer

ECW PRESS

The publication of *Better Medicine* has been generously supported by the Canada Council, the Ontario Arts Council, and the Government of Canada through the Book Publishing Industry Development Program. **Canadä**

Material from "Myths about US Health Care," by David Henderson, is reprinted from *The Joy of Freedom: An Economist's Odyssey* by permission of Reuters Prentice Hall.

NATIONAL LIBRARY OF CANADA CATALOGUING IN PUBLICATION DATA

Gratzer, David
Better medicine: reforming Canadian health care
ISBN 1-55022-505-7
1. Health care reform – Canada. I. Title
RA395.C3G7195 2002   362.1'0971   C2001-903582-9

Typesetting by Yolande Martel.
Cover by Guylaine Régimbald – SOLO DESIGN.
Copyedited by Jodi Lewchuk.
This book is set in Minion and Argo.
Printed by Transcontinental.

Distributed in Canada by General Distribution Services,
325 Humber College Boulevard, Etobicoke, Ontario M9W 7C3.

Distributed in the United States by Independent Publishers Group,
814 North Franklin Street, Chicago, Illinois 60610.

Distributed in Europe by Turnaround Publisher Services, Unit 3,
Olympia Trading Estate, Coburg Road, Wood Green, London N2Z 6T2.

Distributed in Australia and New Zealand by Wakefield Press,
17 Rundle Street (Box 2266), Kent Town, South Australia 5071.

Published by ECW PRESS
Suite 200
2120 Queen Street East,
Toronto, Ontario M4E 1E2.

ecwpress.com

TABLE OF CONTENTS

ACKNOWLEDGEMENTS

Collaborative efforts can be a perilous endeavour. Despite the numerous authors (spread over three countries and two continents), this project proved to be both interesting and entertaining. It was truly a pleasure to work with the contributors. In particular, I would like to thank Michael Bliss for his early and unconditional support — and his reassuring words.

Several people provided valuable advice during the embryonic stages. I am particularly thankful for the suggestions forwarded by Lorne Gunter, Neil Seeman, David Frum, and Patrick Luciani. As with *Code Blue*, my father served an essential and defining role.

I am grateful for the support of the Marigold Foundation, the Donner Canadian Foundation, and the Atlantic Institute for Market Studies.

Jodi Lewchuk did an excellent job editing the manuscript. My publisher, Robert Lecker, was a pleasure to work with. Holly Potter, formerly of ECW Press, taught me much about book publishing.

I would also like to thank my family for their moral support — and Cheryl Wein for tolerating my distracted state.

Of course, the responsibility for any errors within rests with the editor.

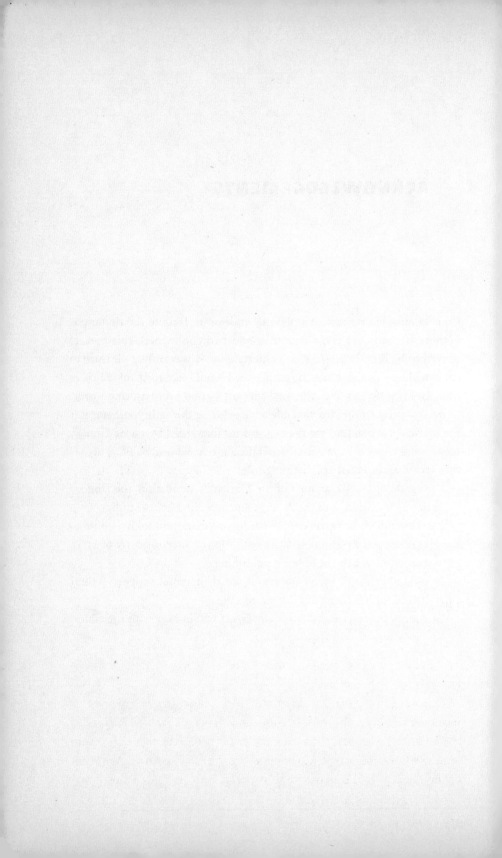

FOREWORD

Canada's health care system has been a subject of intense debate for the last two decades. Beginning in the late 1970s, the federal and provincial governments found that the financial commitment to medicare and other cost-sharing programs was greater than they believed could be afforded. This problem led to "restructuring": closing hospitals and hospital beds, reducing access to various diagnostic programs, and limiting the acquisition of new equipment. These measures, in effect, introduced "rationing by the queue."

Polling over the last decade has consistently shown an escalating concern about the deterioration of services and about the increase in waiting times. (Public angst has grown to the extent that, as noted in an Ekos Research poll commissioned by the federal government last January, the number of supporters for a "two-tiered–private pay competitive system" has increased by 50 percent since 1995.) The public's perception of a faltering system is correct. According to the Organisation for Economic Co-Operation and Development (OECD), Canada rates 12th out of 15 countries for CT scanners, 11th out of 13 for MRIs, and 10th out of 11 for kidney and gallstone breakers. Canada has 2 PET scanners for patients; the United States has 250.[1] Even a nonelective, life-saving treatment such as dialysis for kidney failure is relatively unavailable.[2]

Canada also has a major problem with the supply of health professionals, including nurses and doctors. In 1999, 4,000 fewer students were enrolled in Canada's nursing programs than in 1994.[3] In 2000, one nursing program in British Columbia accepted 33 applicants and turned 300 away. As a result of the nursing (and support staff) shortage, beds have been closed and surgeries cancelled. There are shortages of physicians, both general practitioners and specialists,[4] across Canada.

This crisis in physician resources was in part created when the provincial health ministers adopted some of the recommendations in a report prepared for their deputy ministers.[5] In 1993, the health ministers instituted a 10 percent reduction in entry positions to Canadian medical schools and a 10 percent reduction in post-MD training positions. They optimistically predicted that "population health" measures would significantly reduce the health and medical needs of Canadians. The experience of the last three decades shows, however, that the rate of hip replacements per 1,000 Canadians doubled between 1981–82 and 1996–97, and the rate of knee replacements increased sevenfold over the same period.[6]

For many of us, the major concern is how to improve the performance of the health care system. There is, however, a cadre of health economists and health systems researchers who vigorously defend the status quo of Canada's single-purchaser health care system. They oppose any change to the all-inclusive, first-dollar coverage system. They criticize any form of patient copayments or premiums, any decrease in the scope of coverage, any participation from the private sector, and any different way for Canadians to "draw down" on their health care benefits. They deny evidence that there is impaired access to quality health care and that waiting lists for needed services are long, with people suffering and dying as a result.[7] They also ignore the financial impact of delayed care to individual workers and to Canadian society. They allege that the system needs only more management (especially reform to physician compensation) to cure its ills. Thus, while they talk about "reform," the recommendations promoted by these individuals are merely extensions of the present command-and-control structure. They have consistently accused any who dare to suggest change of acting out of self-interest and greed. They conveniently overlook the notion that labor groups, as well as some in the health systems research community, profit from the contracts they receive to defend the status quo.[8]

The federal and various provincial governments have funded groups to review the Canadian health care system. It appears that these governments have almost always chosen members for these commissions with a view to ensuring a predictable conclusion. Often these individuals move from one review group to another, eliminating the possibility of diverse opinion and alternative considerations.[9]

In short, the command-and-control system characterized by central planning, bureaucratic rule, special interests, and political interference impairs the productivity and responsiveness of our current health care system. Unfortunately, the proposals of our health care "experts" do not offer help.

Better Medicine addresses all of these issues and more importantly, considers what steps need to be taken in order to fix medicare. The contributors, eminent experts in their fields, provide their perspectives on the problems crippling health care in Canada. Seeded throughout are insights into the failure of a single-purchaser system, which lacks the incentives inherent in a competitive market system — incentives that could provide efficient, timely, cost-effective, and high-quality services and care.

The solutions recommended by the contributors are based on economic theory and on the results of experiments undertaken worldwide. The evidence shows that implementing these recommendations would lower the cost and increase the availability of better-quality service. Indeed, to avoid consideration and action on these recommendations would condemn the people of Canada to a continued legacy of "bitter medicine," a fate we do not deserve.

If Canada's health care system is, as its promoters and defenders claim, "the best health care system in the world," why, asks this volume, "isn't a single [Western] country considering a Canada Health Act of its own?"

This book is thoughtful, provocative, and readable. It makes its points clearly and well. It is sure to stimulate debate and should be read by anyone interested in health care — consumers, providers, politicians, bureaucrats, researchers, academics, and policy analysts alike.

— Victor Dirnfeld, MD, FRCPC, DABIM

Past President, Canadian Medical Association
Past President and Past Board of Directors Chair,
British Columbia Medical Association
Richmond, BC, January 2002

NOTES

1. Statistics found in: Organisation for Economic Co-Operation and Development, "Health Data 1999" in *In Search of Sustainability: Prospects for Canada's Health Care System* (Ottawa: CMA, 2000), A34; Heather Sokoloff, "Doctors Demand More High-Tech Cancer Scanners," *National Post*, 6 July 2001, A1, A8; and H.J. Weiler and R.E. Coleman, eds. *PET in Clinical Oncology* (Darmstadt: Steinkopff Verlag Darmstadt Publishers, 2000). With regard to PET scanners, The Institute for Clinical Evaluative

Sciences, in a report prepared for the Ontario Ministry of Health, the Ontario Hospital Association, and the Ontario Medical Association, validated the efficacy, cost effectiveness, and clinical utility of Positron Emission Tomography (PET) for a wide spectrum of cancers, saving patients from having to undergo invasive tests and unnecessary surgery. This explains why the technology is commonly used in Germany, the United Kingdom, Australia, and France.

2. D. Mendelssohn, "Dialysis Delivery in Canada: Can Systemic Shortcomings Cause Complications?" in *Complications of Dialysis — Recognition and Management*, R. Mehta and N. Lameire, eds. (New York: Marcel Dekker, 2000).

3. Canadian Institute of Health Information, *Health Care In Canada* (Ottawa: CIHI, 2001), 50.

4. Including anesthesiologists; cardiologists; ear, nose, and throat surgeons; neurologists; neurosurgeons; orthopedic and general surgeons; radiation oncologists; and radiologists.

5. N.L. Barer and G.L. Stoddart, *Toward Integrated Medical Resource Policies for Canada* (Ottawa: Government of Canada, 1991), 1–6. It should be noted that some have tried to explain the adverse outcome of the above physician reduction policy on the basis that the Barer and Stoddart recommendations were "cherry picked" and not implemented in their totality. These people refuse to recognize that some of these key recommendations would have been impossible to implement. (Take, for example, the directive to substitute nurses for doctors as primary care providers, which is impossible given the national and, in fact, global lack of nurse availability and the international competition for nurses for bedside and specialty unit care. Further, there is the even more fundamental problem of the paucity of evidence for nurses being either as effective or as cost-effective as physicians as primary health care providers and gatekeepers to the health care system.)

6. OECD, "Health Data 1999," A32.

7. J. Sampalis, S. Bookas et al., "Impact of Waiting Time on the Quality of Life of Patients Awaiting Coronary Artery Bypass Grafting," *Canadian Medical Association Journal* 165.4 (21 Aug. 2001): 429–33 and Nancy E. Mayo, Susan C. Scott, Ningyan Shen, James Hanley, Mark S. Goldberg, and Neil MacDonald, "Waiting Time for Breast Cancer Surgery in Quebec," *CMAJ* 164.8 (17 Apr. 2000): 1133–138.

8. Michael Rachlis, Patrick Lewis, Robert G. Evans, and Morris Barer, *Revitalizing Medicare: Shared Problems, Public Solutions* (Vancouver: The Tommy Douglas Institute, 2001), 1–51.

9. Various speakers in the Prime Minister's National Forum media scrum, Feb. 1997; S. Lewis, "Still Here, Still Flawed, Still Wrong: The Case Against the Case for Taxing the Sick," *CMAJ* 159.5 (8 Sept. 1998): 497–99; and Rachlis et al., *Revitalizing Medicare*.

INTRODUCTION

"Sweden is a very socialist nation, but we have always been to the west of the Iron Curtain." So responded Johan Hjertqvist to my question about the legality of private health insurance in his home country.

In politics, there are moments when a comment made in public discussion deeply impresses people — defining moments, if you will. They occur infrequently, perhaps once or twice in a lifetime. In Canada, pundits like to remind us about the Mulroney-Turner exchange ("You, sir, had an option").

But in our personal lives, defining moments — encounters, conversations, or e-mail exchanges that leave a deep impression — are less rare. And on a cool October evening, Hjertqvist's quick, passing comment about health care in his country helped clarify my thinking about health care in my own.

Hjertqvist is a Swedish health care expert and a former deputy mayor. In October 2000, he was in Canada to speak at the Montreal Economic Institute's conference about recent reforms in the Swedish system.

Sweden is a nation dominated by its government. Public spending accounts for roughly 60 percent of the GDP. No wonder: the government is involved in everything from advising adolescent teens on the nuances of physical development to subsidizing and regulating the Lutheran Church. But even in *über*government Sweden, private citizens can buy private health insurance. Indeed, as Hjertqvist's comment implies, only the communists would forbid a person to buy such insurance. The irony, of course, is that in Canada — a country with a much smaller and less intrusive government — private insurance is prohibited. Indeed, the very idea of allowing a private option is opposed by practically every prominent politician, health economist, policy analyst, medical reporter, and administrator.

◆

Successful political and social movements — those that capture the imagination of the citizenry — are rare without leading intellectual proponents:
think of Keynes and Statism, Lévesque and Quebec Separatism, Marx and
Communism. Frequently, however, movements are unable to survive their
main proponents. Despite a multitude of followers, the philosophy of
Objectivism died with Ayn Rand.

Yet there is no easily identifiable figure behind medicare. It is a curiosity
that this 1960s idea, copied in its entirety from another country, would for
so many evolve into the defining characteristic of our nationhood. But if
there is no single individual behind the idea, there is orthodoxy.[1] Medicare
proponents do not quote from a *Das Kapital*-like volume, but they do have
a common argument. There is a nearly uniform view of health care among
our decision-makers and their advisors. It runs something like this: Canada
has the best health care system in the world, an achievement so great that
it is a mark of our civility and citizenship. While problems do exist, they
can be rectified. For this rectification, look to the government to intervene
with greater public spending and better public management. But beware:
Any proposed change to this system based on individual choice and competition would be an "Americanization," and thus disastrous.

This brief summary captures the Majority Opinion of Canada's political class. And, in many ways, we are now at a historic high-water mark in
terms of this Opinion.

The concept of a free-for-all, government-run health care monopoly is
relatively new to Canada. Remember that until about fifteen years ago, extra-
billing and user fees were allowed. But today, practically no political party
— federal or provincial — openly challenges the Majority Opinion. There is
a near homogeneity in the public statements made by government officials.

The Canadian Medical Association and other major lobby groups once
openly debated ideas like private insurance. While the resolutions supporting such options failed, the votes were close. In recent years, however,
members have subscribed to blanket statements, such as the one purport-
ing that "a health care system can't be everything to everybody" (an idea so
vacuous that even the World Health Organization endorses this position).

Health care was the key issue in the last federal election, observed many
experts. But if it was, exactly what sort of debate occurred? On health

policy, the Liberals and the Canadian Alliance sounded remarkably alike. Jean Chrétien's party touted home care and health information, and suggested that high-tech equipment is lacking in the present system. Stockwell Day's party emphasized innovation within the context of the Canada Health Act (read: home care) and favoured increased funding for medicare to support more high-tech equipment and better health information systems.

Indeed, so rigid and ideological has the discussion about medicare become that even the suggestion of change is considered controversial. In spring 2001, Ontario Premier Mike Harris openly contemplated contracting out more services to the private sector. As we shall soon see, this idea is widely accepted in Western Europe, even in countries like Sweden. Still, in Canada, advocating private services — even if they are government funded and regulated with no cost to the patient — is considered an attack on the system.

At the beginning of my first book, *Code Blue: Reviving Canada's Health Care System*, I suggest that the debate over reform is between two groups: the magicians and the spendthrifts. The magicians believe that with just the right combination of government regulations, medicare will miraculously work; the spendthrifts argue that more government money will solve every problem, from the attitude of the grumpiest hospital orderly to the length of the most extreme waiting list for radiation therapy.

In the Introduction of *Code Blue*, I reject both points of view. Magicians and spendthrifts alike believe in a government-run health care system. And while they don't agree on the best way to reform medicare, they basically agree that government action, through more spending or better management, will provide a solution.

At the time, the friction between the magicians and the spendthrifts was quite palpable. Since publication of the book, however, that divide has basically collapsed. The best way to describe the current situation is to plagiarize a good Jefferson line: We are all magicians now; we are all spendthrifts now.[2]

Indeed, the Majority Opinion influences government policy across the land. Every province is dramatically increasing health spending (by an average of 22 percent between 1998 and 2000). Every province is increasing its role in the management of health care. These actions are undertaken, of course, with altruistic motives. But do they represent an effective strategy?

The Majority Opinion certainly seems to think so. Consider, for example, the prescription for better health care that Dr. Carolyn Bennett, a Toronto physician and a Member of Parliament, makes in her book.[3] Dr. Bennett finishes *Kill or Cure?* by advocating increased funding, as well as putting patients first and providing better health information, accountability, and quality. All of these goals are admirable, but they are the same ones health administrators have pursued for three decades. (It's difficult to image that a government would publicly endorse a strategy to deliberately put patients second or make the system less accessible, accountable, or adequate.) What would suddenly make this strategy work now?

Essentially, the history of medicare is a trend toward ever increasing government spending and management. Despite perceptions of deep cuts in the 1990s, health care expenditures today are at an all-time high. Despite arguments that government must "reform" medicare to make it more efficient, government management has never been greater.

When medicare was introduced, the goal was to provide excellent care for all. As quality continues to erode, the Majority Opinion now emphasizes equity. Mr. Smith (who is poor) may wait a year for his cataract surgery, unable to drive a car or watch television, but that's acceptable provided Mr. Jones (who is wealthy) waits six months for his bypass, even though he suffers crushing angina every time he walks up a flight of stairs.

It's not surprising, then, that the Majority Opinion holds sway with our polity, and not necessarily with our public. Certainly, despite the reassuring voice of the experts, Canadians wonder about the quality of care. Early in 2000, Angus Reid (now Ipsos-Reid) surveyed Canadians on the state of medicare: 78 percent of Canadians suggested that the system is "in crisis." In a Canadian Medical Association-commissioned poll in the summer of 2001, people voiced similar dissatisfaction. Asked to grade access to emergency services, a majority of Canadians gave a "C" or an "F," as they did for access to specialist care. On management of health issues, Canadians gave their provincial governments a failing grade.

More surprising still, however, is polling data on the "unthinkable" changes to medicare. In a Maclean's-Global Television poll of 1,400 Canadians, roughly half (47 percent) support a two-tiered system. Support for user fees was even higher: 54 percent of respondents favour the idea.

Interestingly, regional difference has little impact on opinion. Atlantic Canadians endorsed co-payment with almost as much zeal as British Columbians (52 percent and 55 percent, respectively). Saskatchewan, the great hub of prairie socialism, has the highest level of support for user fees, at 69 percent. Only in Ontario did support fall below a majority, but just barely — 48 percent would accept moderate user fees.

Others polls have produced similar results. In the Canadian Medical Association survey, for instance, 57 percent supported user fees. Liberal pollster Michael Marzolini sampled 4,200 citizens in August 2001, finding that a clear majority of Canadians support both user fees and a private insurance option. He noted that when he first asked questions of this kind in 1991, only a small percentage of the public accepted such ideas.

The Majority Opinion, it turns out, is actually a minority opinion. Canadian experts also seem to sense the change in mood. Gone is the rhetoric about Canadians opposing choice or competition. Instead, the experts now speak about our "values" and policies that support those values. (*Toronto Star* columnist James Travers writes, "Canadians understand that a progressive health care system is as much about values as it is about services."[4])

Is the waning public support justified? A quick scan of news items certainly suggests the public is right to have doubts about medicare. Consider some recent stories:

- The head of trauma care at Vancouver's largest hospital announces the facility turns away more cases than any other centre in North America. "This would be unheard of in the United States," he says.[5]

- New Brunswick becomes the seventh province to send cancer patients to the United States for radiation therapy.[6]

- Toronto is rocked by the story of a man who, having endured a heart attack, lies critically ill on a stretcher just outside a hospital unwilling to admit him. The man suffers a second heart attack and is transported to another hospital where he dies. The incident is reported in newspapers the same week a New Brunswick baby dies after being sent to a hospital fifty kilometres from his home; a closer hospital wasn't accepting patients. And these troubling reports are just the latest additions to a growing list: a Winnipeg man dies in an emergency room after waiting for three hours without seeing a doctor; a Vancouver man dies unattended in the ER of a hospital; a Montreal woman passes, unseen by a physician, in a Quebec hospital.

Experts, however, dismiss such stories as sensational journalism or evidence of local problems. ("There aren't any problems when *I* try to get help," is the wonderfully narcissistic observation made so often by media personalities, as though it would be appropriate to dismiss concerns about child poverty by saying, "*My* children aren't poor.") But while the Majority

Opinion denies any serious woes with the system, an expanding body of evidence suggests that quality care is suffering under the current strain.

Those of us actually working in the health care system have no difficulty giving examples. The head of family medicine at a large Montreal hospital says the system is so overwhelmed that emergency surgeries are often delayed. He relates the tale of an elderly man with a broken hip. While his orthopedic surgery was postponed for three days, he developed a blood clot and a potentially life-threatening pulmonary embolism.

In his speech to the Canada Club, Ontario Medical Association President Albert Schumacher neatly described the situation:

> When I began practising medicine nearly twenty years ago, the very idea of waiting for care in Ontario would have seemed far-fetched. How the world has changed — waiting lists have become the norm rather than the exception. They are now a fact of life. Ask anyone who serves on the front lines of the health care system and compare their recent experiences to the way things used to be. . . . People are on waiting lists just to get onto other waiting lists for the treatment they need. So it has come to the point where we have waiting lists to get on waiting lists.[7]

Schumacher went on to describe the situation in his own community: "[In] Windsor, for example, it now takes six months to obtain a hip replacement. Five months to get a CT scan. One of my patients waited more than a year for cardiac surgery. And some of our cancer patients still have to go to the United States for their treatment."

These examples are all anecdotes. But major studies have also suggested that there are problems with the availability and timeliness of care:

- In an annual survey involving more than 2,500 doctors in twelve different specialties, the Fraser Institute found that the total average waiting time from the initial visit to the family doctor through to surgical therapy was sixteen weeks, a significant increase over the last year of the study. In every category, physicians felt waiting times had exceeded "clinically reasonable" delays.[8]

- In the fall of 2000, the Canadian Association of Radiologists released a report suggesting that 63 percent of X-ray equipment is out of date, as is the majority of diagnostic machinery in Canada. One-third of the radiological equipment in the city of Victoria, for example, is over two decades old. (When a hospital there tried to give away one of its ultrasound machines to a local vet, he declined — his own equipment was better.) The Canadian Association of Radiologists then commissioned a legal opinion. Lawyers advised Canadian radiologists to tell patients to "shop around" for facilities with newer equipment (even if it means looking outside Canada), as the quality of care available with the present machines is questionable: "[I]t is imperative that the patient . . . understand the risks and uncertainties associated with the reliability of such . . . examination[s]."[9]

- The Cancer Advocacy Coalition, a patient group based in Toronto, recently released a report on cancer care. It warns that long waiting lists for radiation, coupled with the slow approval of new chemo drugs, have an impact on patient survival. The report includes data on mortality rates, and among the findings is the startling revelation that a person in New Brunswick is twice as likely to die from colorectal cancer as a person in Utah. While the report doesn't adjust for incidence of cancer, comparing similar jurisdictions (which helps to factor out lifestyle and diet issues) still yields surprising results: colorectal cancer mortality rates are 15 percent higher in New Brunswick than in Maine. Responding to critics, the Cancer Advocacy Coalition has released new analysis that includes incidence of disease (which completely factors out lifestyle issues): Canadian provinces rank lower than American states.[10]

- In a five-country survey of health care, the Harvard School of Public Health asked specialists if the quality of care has declined in their region. Sixty-three percent of Canadian specialists responded in the affirmative, the highest percentage of all nations surveyed. When the Harvard researchers looked at waiting times, again Canada fared poorly. In the scenario of a fifty-year-old woman with an irregular breast mass, specialists in Canada responded that she had a 19 percent chance of waiting longer than a month for a biopsy, a higher percentage than in any of the other four countries (in the United States, for example, 90 percent of patients are biopsied within two weeks).[11]

- In a major international study, the Heart & Stroke Foundation of Canada found that Canadian heart attack survivors have a dramatically lower quality of life than their U.S. counterparts. The findings revealed that after twelve months, 31 percent of Canadians rate their health as better than in the month before the cardiac event; in the U.S., 44 percent of survivors feel their health is better. Researchers partly attribute the difference to the availability of angioplasty and bypass surgery south of the forty-ninth parallel. "No question, [Americans] are more aggressive in the early management of heart attacks," observes Dr. Anthony Graham, a Toronto cardiologist.[12]

And there are, of course, many other studies that point in the same direction.[13]

Not that long ago, Canadians could boldly claim that medicare was excellent without pausing to qualify the statement. Today, Canadians wonder about both the quality and timeliness of care. They wonder about what can be done to solve the problem. The Majority Opinion is rigid in its outlook. At a time when the system appears to be crumbling, no talk of individual choice or competition is tolerated. Indeed, the very suggestion is greeted with the charge of "Americanization." But if our political elite won't entertain such an option, why are so many other countries going this route? Consider the developments overseas:

- In Sweden, major health services are being privatized, lowering costs and increasing patient satisfaction.
- German public hospitals are being privatized and within five years, the majority will be in private hands.
- The Australian government recently announced tax incentives for people purchasing private insurance.

Canadians believe that our health care system distinguishes us from the United States. But medicare has grown so rigid that it distinguishes us from *any* Western nation. It is said that plagiarism is the sincerest form of flattery. The Majority Opinion maintains that our approach to health care is superior to any other in the Western world. If that's the case, why the lack of flattery? In all my research, I have never encountered a country presently contemplating a ban on private insurance, the scrapping of user fees, or the termination of extra-billing. The Canada Health Act, portrayed as a model of efficiency and equity, isn't used as a template for legislative reform in any other Western nation.

Finally, there is the question of what the future will bring. The Majority Opinion argues that medicare is in a time of transition, a public policy adolescence. In fact, there is good reason to believe that the stress on our health care system will continue to grow with time as our population ages. If we can't meet today's demand, what will happen when (to borrow a line from columnist George Will) the baby boomers discover arthritis?

◆

We must move beyond the Majority Opinion.

The time has come to think seriously about medicare. This volume attempts to do just that. It combines the efforts of journalists, academics, physicians, and policy analysts in a sober examination of Canada's health policy.

The book is divided into five distinct parts. The seven essays in Parts 1 through 3 consider the past, present, and future of Canadian health care. The two essays in Part 4 put health care into an international context. Finally, the four essays in Part 5 look at ways to reform medicare. Each essay opens with a summary by the editor.

Politically and geographically, the contributors span the spectrum. One author recently contested a Liberal nomination for a provincial by-election while another calls himself a "libertarian." The essayists live in every region of the country, and one even calls Stockholm his home.

The contributors' language is clear and concise. This volume contains no dry academic prose or inscrutable technical terms. A National Newspaper Award (the highest honour in Canadian journalism) recipient details the frustrations of Canada's doctors and nurses. One of the most popular lecture circuit speakers in the country inks a piece on demographics. A McGill economist, recent winner of a major award for humour writing, describes the basics of health economics.

And the contributors aren't simply deft with a pen; they are recognized experts on health care, both in Canada and abroad. One of the most celebrated medical historians in North America traces medicare's history. The Swedish health care expert overseeing Stockholm's privatization project coauthors an investigation of international health reform. A former senior economist with the President's Council of Economic Advisers performs an analysis of the American health care system. And a physician who (informally) advises two provincial governments outlines new reform ideas for Canada.

The book, in brief, is as follows:

Part 1: How We Got Here

Health Care without Hindrance:
Medicare and the Canadian Identity
by Michael Bliss

Professor Michael Bliss writes a political history of medicare. He argues that our obsession with universal health care stems from a modern desire to distinguish ourselves from the Americans. As a result, medicare — once considered a fringe idea — has evolved from a source of public angst into an absolute truth.

Part 2: Surveying the Situation

On the Front Lines
by Margaret Wente

Columnist Margaret Wente focuses on a handful of practising physicians and nurses in this "voices" piece. Through their front line accounts, Wente tackles the unmentionable topics in Canadian health care: queue jumping, excessive waiting times, and provider burnout.

Second Thoughts
by William Orovan

Dr. William Orovan has become one of the country's leading critics of the current health care system, despite the fact that most doctors choose to play a muted role in the health care reform debate. In this one-on-one interview with the editor, Orovan explains his active participation in the movement for change.

Low-Tech, Low-Brow
by Neil Seeman

Neil Seeman explores how the high-tech medical revolution continues to change the face of modern medicine. In particular, Seeman describes many life-saving innovations not available in Canada due to the cost-conscious mentality of the provincial governments.

Five Decades of Observations
by J. Edwin Coffey

Dr. J. Edwin Coffey has been involved in medicine for more than five decades and witnessed first-hand the introduction of medicare and its effects on health care delivery. Drawing on his personal experiences as a family doctor and specialist, Coffey describes his reservations about the quality and sustainability of medicare.

Public System, State Secret
by David Zitner and Brian Lee Crowley

Dr. David Zitner and Dr. Brian Lee Crowley team up to investigate the topics of information, accountability, and transparency within medicare. They discover a system where basic questions cannot be answered, despite bureaucratic commitment to improve health information. Zitner and Crowley explain how medicare's existence as an unregulated monopoly produces information gaps and perverse incentives that undermine the quality and accessibility of care in Canada.

Part 3: Looking Ahead

Population Matters:
Demographics and Health Care in Canada
by David Baxter

Demographer David Baxter has written extensively on the impact of aging demographics. Here, Baxter draws on his extensive body of research to demonstrate how cost pressures on our health care system will worsen as Canada ages, indicating that the current strain is not transient, as many would like to believe.

Part 4: Health Care in an International Context

Myths about U.S. Health Care
by David R. Henderson

Dr. David R. Henderson takes a careful look at health care in the United States and finds that, despite the Canadian perception of radical capitalism, the U.S. system is mired in regulation, government intervention, and bureaucratic meddling. Henderson gets to the root of the *real* problems with U.S. health care, including the uninsured and third party payment.

Accessible, High-Quality, and Cost-Effective Health Care:
A Public or Private Matter?
by Cynthia Ramsay

Health economist Cynthia Ramsay provides an international perspective on health care through a discussion of various health care systems that goes beyond simplistic statistics like infant mortality rates. Ramsay includes findings from her new international comparison study.

Part 5: Up from Stalemate

Thirty-Million-Tier is Near
by William Watson

Economist William Watson discusses the "truths" of Canadian health care: the health care market is a failure, user fees don't work, profit-seeking increases prices, etc. Watson thoughtfully dismisses these assertions and provides Health Economics 101, a crash course in an alternative to today's central planning approach.

Health Reform Abroad
by Carl Irvine, Johan Hjertqvist, and David Gratzer

Economist Carl Irvine and health expert Johan Hjertqvist join me in an evaluation of health reforms in other countries, specifically the new private-public partnership trend in Sweden and the United Kingdom. We discover that many of the ideas considered radical here in Canada (private insurance, user fees, etc.) are common abroad.

Making Health Spending Work
by Fred McMahon and Martin Zelder

Policy analyst Fred McMahon and Dr. Martin Zelder debunk the current idea that more money will solve medicare's woes. McMahon and Zelder use data from the 1990s to show that perverse incentives within the system create a situation in which spending is at an all-time high while waiting lists are longer than ever. They then argue for replacing these incentives through an overhaul in medicare's funding.

The ABCs of MSAs
by David Gratzer

I outline the structural problems with medicare and a potential solution: the introduction of individual choice and provider competition through medical savings accounts. Based on the experience of countries like Singapore, the United States, South Africa, and China with both public and private MSAs, I suggest that it is possible to maintain universality and sustainability in our medicare system without waiting lists.

NOTES

1. A similar observation is made about Aboriginal public policy in Tom Flanagan's Donner Prize-winning book, *First Nations? Second Thoughts* (Montreal: McGill-Queen's University Press, 2000).
2. A slight exception to this development is the final report of Saskatchewan's Commission on Medicare, written by former Deputy Minister Kenneth Fyke. Originally commissioned by then Premier Roy Romanow, the document probably foreshadows the findings of Romanow's Federal Commission, due to report in November 2002.

    The report is very critical of the present system, stating that "Essentially the system pays for activity and is indifferent to result." Unlike most Canadian surveys of medicare, the final report avoids the usual America bashing: "[I]t is inconceivable that American health care organizations pay less attention to quality and service than ours given their competitive insurance structure and their litigation-friendly jurisdiction. In fact, given that quality has more funding and champions in the United States than in Canada, it is likely that, if anything, our circumstances are worse."

Still, despite such strong criticism of the status quo and the argument that more money will not resolve our woes, Fyke recommends a variety of magician-like prescriptions: fewer regional health boards, an annual report, a new committee to oversee quality, and primary care "reform." See The Commission on Medicare, *Caring for Medicare: Sustaining a Quality System* (Regina: Government of Saskatchewan, 2000).

3. Carolyn Bennett and Rick Archbold, *Kill or Cure? How Canadians Can Remake Their Health Care System* (Toronto: HarperCollins Publishers Ltd., 2000).

4. James Travers, "Don't Expect Prescription for User Fees," *Toronto Star*, 28 June 2001, A27.

5. Pamela Fayerman, "Lack of Beds Forces VGH to Reject Trauma Patients: Vancouver's High Level of Diversion 'Unheard of in North America,'" *Vancouver Sun*, 11 Oct. 2000, A1.

6. Carol McLeod, "N.B. Radiology Patients Being Sent to Maine," *Medical Post* 36 (12 Sept. 2000): 5.

7. Dr. Albert Schumacher, "A Prescription for Health Care Reform: From Myth to Dialogue to Solutions," address to the Canada Club, Toronto, ON, 19 Mar. 2001.

8. Michael Walker with Greg Wilson, *Waiting Your Turn: Hospital Waiting Lists in Canada*, 11th ed. (Vancouver: The Fraser Institute, 2000), 49–50.

9. Special Ministerial Briefing, *Outdated Radiology Equipment: A Diagnostic Crisis* (Saint-Laurent: Canadian Association of Radiologists, 2000), 7.

10. The full study can be found at www.canceradvocacycoalition.com. The Coalition's findings are based on the North American Association of Central Cancer Registries, Colon and Rectal Cancer (Male), Mortality, Mortality/Incidence, and Incidence Rates in Canada and the United States, 1993–97.

11. Robert J. Blendon, Cathy Schoen, Karen Donelan, Robin Osborn, Catherine M. DesRoches, Kimberly Scoles, Karen Davis, Katherine Binns, and Kinga Zapert, "Physicians' Views on Quality of Care: A Five-Country Comparison," *Health Affairs* 20 (May/June 2001): 233–43.

12. Brad Evenson, "Cardiac Care Better in U.S., Study Shows: Fewer Are Dying, but Canadian Heart Attack Patients Have Poorer Quality of Life," *National Post*, 8 Feb. 2001, A4.

13. In a major study of waiting time for breast surgery in Quebec, Nancy Mayo et al. reviewed 29,606 patient cases between 1992 and 1998. They found that the median waiting time between diagnosis and the OR rose from twenty-nine days in 1992 to forty-two days in 1998, an increase of 37 percent. More alarming was that the number of patients waiting longer than ninety days rose from 11 percent to 17 percent. See Nancy E. Mayo, Susan C. Scott, Ningyan Shen, James Hanley, Mark S. Goldberg, and Neil MacDonald, "Waiting Time for Breast Cancer Surgery in Quebec," *Canadian Medical Association Journal* 164 (2001): 1133–1138.

The Manitoba Centre for Health Policy and Evaluation did an audit of surgical waiting times in Winnipeg. Between 1991 and 1997, the authors found "no general recent increase in waiting times, and that for some services waits have decreased." But there is a limitation to the study: it looked only at the interval between surgical consultation and the operation. Additionally, the sample was small, confined to eight non-urgent surgeries in Winnipeg. The conclusion was heralded by the Majority Opinion as evidence that medicare's problems have been greatly exaggerated (The Tommy Douglas Institute, for example, cited this work in a recent paper).

The Manitoba Centre, however, recently updated the study to cover two more years and found waiting times have increased for seven out of the eight procedures reviewed. The wait for varicose vein removal, for example, is up by 50 percent. Waits for more medically significant surgeries — breast tumour removal and carotid endarterectomies — also show increases. The Manitoba authors suggest the trend is "of concern." See Carolyn De Coster, Leonard MacWilliam, and Randy Walld, "Waiting Times for Surgery: 1997/98 and 1998/99 Update," audit prepared by the Manitoba Centre for Health Policy and Evaluation, Nov. 2000.

PART 1

HOW WE GOT HERE

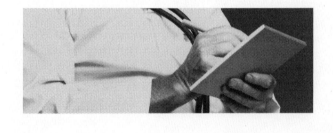

HEALTH CARE WITHOUT HINDRANCE: MEDICARE AND THE CANADIAN IDENTITY

Michael Bliss

For many politicians, health economists, and policy analysts, medicare has become intertwined with our very identity as a nation. But this identification lacks historic context and perspective, as made clear by this sweeping essay in which Professor Michael Bliss describes the evolution of Canadian health care.

The widespread acceptance and implementation of national health insurance is a modern idea. As Bliss observes, health care wasn't even discussed at the time of Confederation. For much of Canada's early history, state involvement in health care remained a fringe idea. Only after World War II did interest in a national initiative grow. While delayed by provincial resistance, large-scale federal involvement started with hospital insurance in 1958.

In the 1960s, Bliss notes that "There was a widespread belief — rooted in the command economy of wartime and in politicians' and policy makers' suspicion of the marketplace (and reinforced by their not inconsiderable hubris) — that in most areas of life, governments had a better capacity than the private sector to plan, organize, and allocate resources." This zeal for government intervention, coupled with a desire for policies that distinguish us from our American neighbours, led to the Pearson government's decision to expand the experiment. National insurance was thus introduced in the late 1960s. Physician opting-out and extra-billing, however, were still allowed.

What followed was the golden age of Canadian medicare. The better Canadian way was "an expression of the caring collective values that were said . . . to flow from the very nature of the country itself." Soon, however, the golden age passed and health insurance became "hellishly expensive," due to two main factors: (1) medical innovation and rising patient expectations and (2) elimination of direct payment. As Bliss points out, the offer of "all sorts of medical and hospital services without requiring direct payment was a recipe for huge increases in the use and abuse of the system by both producers and consumers." Many physicians opted out.

In response, the House of Commons ushered in a second major experiment with national insurance. With the Canada Health Act of 1984, the federal government effectively outlawed private medical and hospital practice and a legislated monopoly became the order of the day. But problems persisted. As with other socialist models, Bliss notes that when you "remove an industry from market conditions, replace price signalling with administrative fiat, [and] outlaw competition . . . you create the classic conditions for inefficiency, declining productivity, and gradually increasing consumer dissatisfaction."

As such, Bliss describes the present day problems not, like some, as the result of recent meddling by local politicians, but rather as the end result of increasingly aggressive government measures to control patients and providers. Bliss concludes by pointing out that at the end of the twentieth century, "The notion that one particular approach to health care was integral to the Canadian identity began to seem increasingly anachronistic." And it will continue to seem that way.

How deeply embedded is universal medicare in the Canadian experience? Does it express our core values as a society? To what extent does it flow from or shape our identity? How malleable has it been? How malleable can it be?

In the following sketch of Canada's history with health insurance, I argue that the country's approach to medicare grew out of a set of particular historical circumstances relating to the evolution of our approaches to health care and the welfare state.[1] There has not been a single Canadian approach to universal health care. Rather, there have been two major experiments with universal health insurance for Canadians: the plan initiated by the Pearson government in the mid-1960s and the Canada Health Act system put in place by the Trudeau government in 1984.

Given the extent and complexity of the Canadian experience since Confederation, the increasing diversity and pluralism of the country at the end of the twentieth century, the rapidly changing Canadian attitudes and interests in the realm of health care, and the shortcomings of the Canadian health insurance system, it defies rationality to equate a particular set of

Canada Health Act constraints imposed by Ottawa with the preservation of the Canadian identity. It makes much more sense to suggest that at the beginning of the twenty-first century, the ideological rigidity of those who see the Canada Health Act as set in Canadian stone has become a hindrance to health care reform and to the country's capacity to adjust to the continuing challenges of the modern world.

◆

Health insurance has comparatively shallow roots in the communities that in 1867 came together to found the Dominion of Canada, as there was effectively no recognizable form of health insurance in the nineteenth century. The provision of health care was simply not a priority for the Fathers of Confederation. Indeed, unlike education, it was not discussed at all. The British North America Act, still the governing document of Canada's constitution, does not even contain the word "health." It has since been deemed by the courts to assign health matters — except for quarantine and marine hospitals — to the provinces. In the raw, root-hog-or-die society of early Canada, hospitals were charities for the indigent to which doctors donated as much of their time and talent as they could muster. Physicians billed their private patients for services rendered, and collected these bills as best they could. The one rudimentary form of health "insurance" came with membership in fraternal or benevolent societies, through which the working poor could, in effect, prepay their funerals. It was also not uncommon for such societies, as well as for corporations mobilizing large numbers of workers in timber camps and other frontier activities, to hire physicians on a contract basis to provide medical services. For one hundred dollars a year, or perhaps fifty cents a head, the doc would look after sick loggers.

The modern era of state involvement in health insurance began in Germany in 1883, with Chancellor Otto von Bismarck's broad scheme of social insurance aimed at cementing the loyalty of the working classes. In 1911, Great Britain launched a system of national health insurance rooted in the contracting experience, where physicians were paid capitation fees for providing services to the needy. Although there was desultory interest in Canada in some of these schemes, the predominant sense before World War I (1914–18) was that a young, hard, prosperous North American country was relatively insulated from the worst of old-world problems and did not need old-world policies. The national symbol of Canada at the beginning of the twentieth century was a tough, sleeves-rolled-up Johnny Canuck, cut from hardy pioneer stock, busy logging and making railways and clearing land and playing hockey and getting ready by 1914 to volunteer to fight the Huns in France. The idea of somebody providing unemployment insurance, a pension, or health insurance for Johnny, or for his good-looking and wholesome little sister, Jane, seemed preposterous. Judging by its real roots, health insurance had more to do with European countries' sense of identity than with Canada's.

After the years of war and slaughter that shook the foundations of western civilization, the idea of protecting victims and the powerless came into vogue. In 1919, before there was any significant party to its left, the Liberal Party of Canada adopted a platform that called for extensive social welfare policies, including a scheme for national medical insurance. This enthusiasm melted in the glow of late 1920s' prosperity and early concerns about constitutional problems, only to be spectacularly revived during the Great Depression of the 1930s. Through those grim years, *someone* had to bear the cost of providing health care services to very large numbers of indigent Canadians.

Canadians' desire for access to health care services increased steadily as medical diagnosis and treatment became routinely more effective. Canadians wanted to be able to visit doctors and use modern hospitals. In what has been called "the health century," health care was becoming more and more important in everyday life. Doctors, the private citizens who had traditionally been expected to provide free health care services, were among the leaders in discussing health insurance. By the late 1930s, groups of physicians were pioneering in private health insurance through such plans as Associated Medical Services and Physicians' Services Incorporated. Moreover, Canada's first doctors' strike had taken place in Winnipeg in 1933; it had been an attempt to force the city's government to accept responsibility for paying for medical services needed by the impoverished.

After the Depression, in the egalitarian climate of World War II, it became conventional wisdom to suggest that Canada follow European countries and the United States (which had initiated social security in 1935) in the creation of a modern "welfare state." Both patients and physicians were drawn to the theoretical attractiveness of some kind of system of national health insurance as part of a complete social safety net. As an Ontario family doctor put the issue in 1944, "Every day I see patients who are getting inadequate medical service, both diagnostic and curative, because they are unable to pay for it, or if they do pay they are left with insufficient money to provide a decent standard of living. Every such case is a demand, even though usually unexpressed, for some form of health insurance."

Only the state seemed to have the resources to organize and support health insurance for populations containing large numbers of relatively poor citizens who would have trouble paying premiums. In 1942, the president of the Winnipeg Medical Society said, "The socialization of medicine is coming as surely as tomorrow's dawn. It is the natural result of public demand for adequate, complete medical service."

By the end of World War II, the Liberal government in Ottawa had become fully committed to the welfare state. It had launched national unemployment insurance in 1941, brought in family allowances or "baby bonuses" in 1945, and introduced universal old age pensions in 1951. It was in 1945 that the government of Canada hoped to proceed with a program of national health insurance.

It found that stakeholder support was very soft. A number of the provinces — notably Alberta, Ontario, and Quebec — were reluctant to see Ottawa intrude further into their constitutional jurisdiction. The medical profession began to worry about the implications of state-dominated health care funding for physician and patient autonomy (similar concerns had undercut proposals for socialized medicine in the United States). Ottawa itself began to have second thoughts and backed off from the idea of a comprehensive approach to begin a more targeted strategy of expanding its involvement in health care through offering conditional grants to the provinces to deal with designated problems of disease control.

But popular interest in being insured against health costs continued to increase. Many Canadians were envious, for example, of the apparent health care security the citizens of Great Britain enjoyed after their country's introduction of full National Health Insurance in 1948. The depression-born Canadian left-wing political party, the Co-operative Commonwealth Federation (CCF), became increasingly interested in advocating socialized medicine — the term was used constantly and proudly — on the British model. In the meantime, private insurers, led by the doctors' groups, were expanding their health offerings and enrolling many new customers. By the 1950s and 1960s, Canadians could choose from a wide variety of medical and hospital plans. By the mid-1960s, physicians' groups had banded together under the umbrella of Trans-Canada Medical Services and could offer something close to national coverage.

There was no golden age of private health insurance in Canada. Carriers and their clients quickly became enmeshed in the complex problems of risk assessment, terms of coverage, and fee negotiations. First-dollar coverage (eliminating any charge to the user) was very popular — the doctors' plans all offered it — but it was apparent that very large numbers of Canadians thought they could not afford the premiums on even basic insurance coverage. And the state would still have to look after the indigent, whatever the definition of that term might be. Most provincial governments, led by Alberta and Ontario, concluded that they could best fulfill their responsibilities by offering either subsidies or special backup insurance, as a welfare measure, to those who could not afford private insurance. On the other hand, the lobby for socialized medicine argued that governments ought to dispense altogether with invidious means-testing, and offer universal, compulsory coverage to bypass the risk assessment problem and keep administrative costs to a minimum.

The CCF government of Saskatchewan, first elected in 1944, led other jurisdictions in introducing health insurance, which began with hospital insurance in 1945–47. Other provinces gradually followed and in 1958, Ottawa introduced a national program based on conditional grants (the courts had determined that Ottawa could constitutionally offer money to the provinces to be spent according to the conditions Ottawa itself imposed). As such, hospital insurance arrived in Canada without major controversy.

But then Saskatchewan introduced universal medical coverage in 1962, prompting a majority of the province's physicians to withdraw their services. The traumatic Saskatchewan doctors' strike lasted twenty-three days — the province's socialist government brought in strikebreaking physicians from Great Britain — and ended in a draw. Doctors retained the right to opt out of the government scheme (that is, to bill patients directly), and to bill at rates higher than for which patients would be indemnified (that is, to "extra-bill"). The general principle of fee-for-service payment was also retained, and the guarantee of a patient's freedom of choice enunciated. (Contract medicine [also known as rostered or capitation medicine] had always been unpopular in North America; the leading example of a contract system, Britain's National Health Service [NHS], was particularly unpopular with physicians and due to an image of deteriorating quality, was losing appeal with well-to-do Canadian patients.)

In the 1960s, Canadians' willingness to experiment with social/socialized policy initiatives in all fields reached its apogee. It was a very prosperous decade, characterized by steadily rising tax revenues for most governments. There was a widespread belief — rooted in the command economy of wartime and in politicians' and policy makers' suspicion of the marketplace (and reinforced by their not inconsiderable hubris) — that in most areas of life, governments had a better capacity than the private sector to plan, organize, and allocate resources. The Communist/Socialist ideal that there should be a social equality greater than the one capitalism seemed to provide had a widespread appeal in Canada and many other Western countries, even if Communism itself was thought a dubious model.

The capitalist United States also seemed a dubious, even menacing, model to Canadians in the 1960s. It seemed particularly important in an age of rising Canadian self-confidence and national assertiveness to choose policies that would help distinguish the country from market-oriented, anti-Communist, world-dominating America. So when, for example, the Cuban revolutionary Fidel Castro declared himself a Communist and U.S.-Cuban ties were abruptly snapped, Canadians continued to recognize and trade with Moscow's newest acolyte. Many left-of-centre Canadians were particularly impressed by the Castro government's initiatives in state-organized health care. The Americans might despise everything connected with the Castro regime, but socialized medicine did not seem to present any terrors for either the Cuban or the Canadian people. And since Canada's socially democratic mother country (admittedly a bit of an aging dowager) had pioneered with the NHS in the 1940s, there was also the comforting thought that state health insurance was a way of reaffirming Canada's basically British identity.

During the prime ministership of Lester Pearson (1963–68), the Ottawa Liberals continued to expand Canada's welfare state by implementing the compulsory Canada Pension Plan. Some provinces socialized automobile insurance. There was even talk of great schemes to eliminate college tuition and to give Canadians a guaranteed annual income. In this climate of happy optimism, the Pearson government also decided that the time had come to initiate national health insurance or "medicare" as it is now known, using the term coined in the United States (as with their currency, their accents, and their preference for baseball and many other American pastimes, Canadians' sense of continental practicality continued to temper their desire to be different). Ottawa's inclination to act was powerfully reinforced by the 1964 report of its Royal Commission on Health Services, which recommended that "as a nation we now take the necessary legislative, organizational and financial decisions to make all the fruits of the health sciences available to all our residents without hindrance of any kind."

The Pearson government announced in 1965 that it proposed to pay half the cost of provincial medicare plans that met four criteria: (1) comprehensive coverage (of necessary medical and hospital costs; the Hall Commission envisaged adding dental and drug coverage), (2) portability across Canada, (3) public administration (there would be no role for the private insurers), and (4) universality. Physician opting-out and extra-billing would be allowed, albeit reluctantly and with foreboding. Against the objections of several provinces and the medical profession in general, national medicare was approved in 1966 on a 177-2 vote in the House of Commons. Implementation began in 1968. With varying degrees of resistance and bitterness, the provinces adjusted their insurance plans to meet Ottawa's conditions. Private insurers had to leave the business.

✦

A brief but very important golden age of Canadian medicare followed. Ordinary Canadians were delighted with the apparent elimination of doctor and hospital bills. Health care was free (well, not quite, as some provinces continued to charge premiums for their coverage even though these premiums were low and eventually eliminated in most cases). But doctors were also delighted because they got fully paid and had no more unremunerative charity cases and no more bills to collect — except the big bill from governments.

Socialized medicine seemed to be working in everyone's interests. In particular, it seemed to be working far, far better than the anarchic mix of health insurance schemes (mostly private and market-driven) in the United States. No wonder Liberal politicians and other medicare supporters boasted of the Canadian way in health care. The better Canadian way, socialized medicine, would be a beacon to the United States — indeed a beacon to the world — an expression of the caring, collective values that were said in those few bright years to flow from the very nature of Canada itself.

Except that health insurance became hellishly expensive. The dynamic of medical innovation and constantly rising patient expectations would have meant relentless cost increases anyway. Throw in the fact that offering all sorts of medical and hospital services without requiring direct payment was a recipe for huge increases in the use and abuse of the system by both

producers and consumers. Like insurers everywhere, Canadian governments found themselves in an endless struggle to contain health care costs,
which in most years rose far faster than the GNP.

The 1970s were plagued by inflation, uneven economic growth, and a
nagging sense that the Camelot years of Canadian social welfare initiatives
were over. Desperate provincial ministries of health tried to redirect spending from therapy to prevention, tried to generate administrative savings
through more direct controls and incentives (especially in hospital care),
and made determined efforts to hold the line on fees paid to doctors and
nurses, who became more disgruntled the more they were squeezed. The
senior and controlling "partner" in health insurance, Ottawa, limited its
liabilities by moving from open-ended cost sharing to specific block grants,
while offering provinces the option of increased taxing leeway.

The endless financial problems led both physicians and some provincial
governments to consider bringing new money into the system through
extra-billing. By the end of the 1970s, large numbers of physicians — particularly specialists — were choosing to opt out of medicare and bill their
patients directly at fees of their own choosing; the patients could get partially reimbursed from the government plans. Provincial governments were
also considering introducing user or deterrent fees. In 1981, the Canadian
Medical Association called for the "demonopolization" of medicare, arguing
that the problem was not extra-billing, but state underfunding.

By 1983, in an atmosphere of general acrimony about health care costs,
opting out in some regions and provinces had become so widespread that it
was impossible for many thousands of Canadians to find "opted-in" providers. The incidence of low-income Canadians being subjected to extra-billing
was increasing. Alberta was proposing to introduce a hospital user fee of
twenty dollars a day. In fact, the original Canadian medicare system was
collapsing from the state's (and taxpayers') reluctance to meet ever rising
costs through the tax system. Socialized medicine was heading inexorably
in the direction of reprivatization.

With public opinion strongly in support of medicare and against extra-
billing, the Trudeau government moved to buttress state health insurance.
It implemented what might be called the "resocialization" of Canadian
medicare through the Canada Health Act, which was passed unanimously
in the House of Commons on April 9, 1984 and became effective on July 1.
As written, the Canada Health Act denies federal support to provinces that
allow extra-billing within their insurance schemes and effectively forbids

private or opted-out practitioners from billing beyond provincially mandated fee schedules. This action was taken in the name of "accessibility," a new principle that was written into the Act.

With passage of the Canada Health Act, the state had inaugurated the second era of Canadian medicare by effectively outlawing private medical and hospital practice. It was true that private medicine would still survive — indeed come to flourish — through the provision of fringe, alternative, and unlisted services. But the public health insurance system, covering core medical and hospital care, was now guaranteed survival, not on its own merits through competition with the private sector — as had been the case for generations in most provinces with, say, education — but through the mechanism of a legislated monopoly. Provinces that did not agree with Ottawa's approach to health care funding again had no realistic choice: the noncompliance costs to their treasuries and taxpayers would be too great. The Canadian public, on the other hand, was unconcerned about anything beyond the promise that medicare was being preserved. Deep physician outrage at losing control of personal freedom, of professional income, and possibly of methods of practice, resulted in a particularly bitter doctors' strike against Ontario's compliance legislation in 1986. It failed. One of the unforeseen consequences of Canadian federalism was the way it facilitated dividing and conquering the medical profession.

In the Canada Health Act era, the cost containment struggle on the part of insurers continued. Cadres of health care bureaucrats and their hired help struggled to manage the system in the context of continual innovation, sharp debate about priorities (including movements toward ambulatory care, hospital restructuring, and reliance on community and home care), fee disputes with the professionals, rising patient expectations, and the unyielding (if poorly understood) logic that success in health care only postpones illness. With private sector alternatives and safety valves removed from the system, however, there was at once more scope for direct control by governments and less leeway for physician and patient manoeuvrability or flexibility.

The legislated single-payer monopoly on the provision of medical and hospital services and consequent infringements on personal and professional liberty were now justified on egalitarian grounds: all Canadians had equal access to the health care system; no one could "jump the queue" by buying health care privately and unlike the United States, Canada offered a single tier of service. Legislated equality in health care (with only a few

quietly permitted loopholes, such as special VIP care for Members of Parliament) was the Canadian way, the very essence of the country's values,
part of the Canadian identity. If you did not agree with these propositions,
the inference would be that your Canadianism was suspect.

If the state monopoly had worked, if governments had been able to
deliver on the 1964 promise of universal access to health care "without hindrance of any kind," the Canada Health Act system might have been seen
by the rest of the world as a distinctively Canadian contribution to health
care. The world might have copied Canada. Even the Americans might
have copied Canada. The trouble was (as most students of monopolistic
behaviour, planned or command economies, or elementary market economics could have forecast) that the Canadian system did not work very well.
By the 1980s, the whole of the Western world had come to appreciate the
flaws of socialist and dirigiste economic management: remove an industry
from market conditions, replace price signalling with administrative fiat,
outlaw competition, and you create the classic conditions for inefficiency,
declining productivity, and gradually increasing consumer dissatisfaction.
Not a single country anywhere copied the flawed Canadian "model."

The whole world was changing. In the 1980s, the historic Communist
experiment collapsed: the Soviet Empire disappeared, China liberalized,
and only North Korea and Cuba hung on as increasingly impoverished
anachronisms, with support for the latter country still a pillar and proof of
Canada's independent foreign policy. Areas of state socialism in democratic
countries were exposed as costly and inefficient. Virtually all Western
countries moved to deregulate their economies and to dismantle bloated
state-owned companies.

In Canada, for example, such dinosaur-like icons as Air Canada, Canadian
National Railways, and Petro-Canada — all of which had been repeatedly
trumpeted as examples of Canadian distinctiveness and excellence — were
privatized. In many countries the welfare state itself began to contract. Retirement saving, for example, no longer seemed most effectively done
through state pension plans. Universal income supplements, such as
Canada's old family allowances, were replaced by programs targeted to
real need. The state would continue to help those who could not help
themselves, but it did not have to dole out benefits to everyone as a matter
of right.

During this era of change, the Canada Health Act continued to be a
sacred Canadian cow. Even as governments wielded their monopoly pow-

ers ruthlessly in health care — curbing the output of physicians and nurses, closing community hospitals by administrative decree, and in Ottawa's case, slashing its grants to the provinces by billions of dollars — citizen and physician concerns were met by slogans and clichés about the Canadian identity, the awfulness of health care in the United States, and the atrocities of a two-tiered system. Even so, public support for the Canada Health Act system began to wither as resource constraints collided with constantly rising expectations to produce health care horror stories and growing skepticism in the media. (One of the most fascinating aspects of the evolving Canadian health care debate relates to changes in journalists' and editorial coverage. From the 1960s through the 1980s, the Canadian media had been remarkably uncritical — was often even an unprofessional cheerleader — of the government programs. In the 1990s, this unchecked approval gradually began to change.)

Canadians themselves found their attitudes and personal values regarding governments and health care changing. The baby boom generation and its offspring were far less deferential to authority and more impatient for results. They were less inclined than earlier generations to tolerate queues, second-rate service, and excuses. As health care workers knew, in an age of patient empowerment that included access to the Internet, Canadians became more insistent on taking responsibility for their own health care decisions. The lack of choice under the Canada Health Act system, the sense that the health care was in the hands of an unaccountable bureaucratic/political elite, and the realization that its managerial decisions were inefficient and divorced from the real health care marketplace began to emerge as key issues for the twenty-first century agenda.

The notion that one particular approach to health care was integral to the Canadian identity began to seem increasingly anachronistic. Aside from the weak historical foundation for the argument (as we have seen, medicare was a healthy centrepiece of Canadian policy for only a few years) it was a simple fact that Canada, Canadian values, and Canadian health care needs were in constant flux. The idea of defining the country and its people by a time- and culture-bound set of policies or symbols — be it a national policy of protective tariffs, a national monopoly of broadcast outlets by CBC, national retailing through the T. Eaton catalogue, or national sport dominated by the Montreal Canadiens hockey team — came to feel increasingly outmoded. In general, as Canadian society became more diverse and pluralistic in every respect, the very notion of an "identity," of insistence that Canadianism involved acceptance of a special socio-political agenda, began to seem narrow and stultifying and offensive.

In Canada's 2000 election campaign, the opposition parties still did not quite dare to demand comprehensive reform to the Canada Health Act. But midway through the campaign, as the Chrétien Liberals blustered about stopping all breaches to the Canada Health Act, it was revealed that card-carrying Liberals were among the backers of the private MRI clinics that had opened in several Canadian provinces to supply prompt diagnostic service. In winter 2001, the public and the media gave short shrift to a report from the Tommy Douglas Institute suggesting that changes to the Canada Health Act would threaten the Canadian identity and were not needed.

✦

Today, like people everywhere in the modern world, Canadians deeply believe in excellence and accessibility in health care. They probably still share much of the idealism of their 1960s forebears who wanted Canada to have a system that would give its people access to hospital and medical care "without hindrance of any kind." But the country has changed. Health care has changed. Canadians have changed. The world has changed. The monopolistic system created by the Canada Health Act, once seen as part of the solution to the problems of public health insurance, has become part of the problem, part of the hindrance citizens face in trying to develop for themselves and their children the best possible health care system.

NOTE

1. A general note on sources: Although there is a vast and scattered literature on aspects of the history of Canadian health care, it has not been drawn together in readily accessible book-length form. The two classic books on the coming of Canadian health insurance remain Malcolm G. Taylor, *Health Insurance and Canadian Public Policy: The Seven Decisions that Created the Canadian Health Insurance System* (Montreal: McGill-Queen's University Press, 1979) and C. David Naylor, *Private Practice, Public Payment: Canadian Medicine and the Politics of Health Insurance* (Montreal: McGill-Queen's University Press, 1986). A handy overview of health insurance issues in the Pearson years can be found in J. L. Granatstein, *Canada 1957–1967: The Years of Uncertainty and Innovation* (Toronto: McClelland & Stewart, 1986). There is a particularly useful historical overview of the coming of the Canada Health Act in Gwendolyn Gray, *Federalism and Health Policy: The Development of Health Systems in Canada and Australia* (Toronto: University of Toronto Press, 1991).

PART 2

SURVEYING THE SITUATION

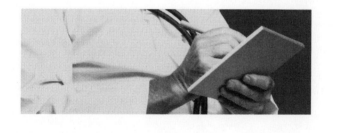

ON THE FRONT LINES

Margaret Wente

Increasingly, Canadians are aware of medicare's shortcomings. A journalist friend recently told me of his good luck: he had a heart attack in Haiti. Why good luck? "Because they air-evacuated me to Florida," he observed. Within three hours, he received an angiography. "I may have been so lucky in Canada, but odds are I would have been treated more conservatively." As noted in the Introduction, the results of a major study done by the Heart & Stroke Foundation of Canada support his view. Patients south of the border (and include in that category the poorest of the poor on Medicare) get better cardiac care than is available in this country.

But relatively little attention is paid to those working on the front lines. We know the patients are frustrated. What about the providers? Margaret Wente, a veteran journalist, observes, "Over the past couple of years, I've written many columns in the *Globe and Mail* about Canada's deteriorating health care system. Nothing has struck me more forcefully than the toll it's taking on its professionals — the nurses, doctors, and hospital administrators who are trying to keep it stuck together with chewing gum and bailing wire. They will say what the politicians will not: The status quo cannot be sustained."

In this "voices" essay, Wente describes the frustration and angst of the men and women working in the system. She takes us on a tour of Toronto's St. Joseph's Emergency Room with Dr. Harry Zeit, where she discovers a "rabbit warren of dark and dingy rooms with ancient beat-up furniture." We meet Dr. Keith MacLeod, an obstetrician in the underserviced community of Windsor, whose caseload is four- or fivefold higher than that of his counterparts in Detroit. "If we had our volumes and their fees," MacLeod notes, "we'd all be as rich as Bill Gates." And then there is Edmonton nurse

Christine Peterson, a "casual worker": always on call, always armed with a pager, and in possession of no job security.

Wente not only describes the frustrations of the system, but its insanity. She talks to Dr. Arnold Aberman, past dean of the University of Toronto's Faculty of Medicine, who was "one of the most popular guys in town. Everyone called him to try to beat the queue." The callers included an assistant deputy minister of health. Dr. Mo Watanabe, the former dean of the University of Calgary's medical school, explains the extent to which Canada suffers from a physician shortage and how this problem is the result of government action.

Through her sixteen vignettes, Wente covers the great unmentionable topics of health care: queue jumping, excessive waiting times, provider burnout, aged equipment, and the politicization of health administration. Wente meticulously catalogues the views of people working under medicare and in doing so, makes a weighty indictment against the system itself.

Not *ER*

Early in 2000, I got an e-mail from an emergency room doctor named Harry Zeit. It was a cry from the heart. He described a health care system that is under great stress, staffed by people who've been stretched too far for too long. He invited me to take a tour of his emergency room with him, and so I did.

I quickly learned that life in the ER bears no resemblance at all to life on *ER*. *ER*, the show, has a large cast of doctors. But Harry Zeit works all alone. He handles the night shift at St. Joseph's, one of the biggest hospitals in downtown Toronto. "You're not really in control here," he told me. Every time he goes to work, he knows he probably won't be able to give people the medical care they deserve.

ER, the show, is well equipped with nurses, beds, and examination tables. Dr. Zeit's ER is a rabbit warren of dark and dingy rooms with ancient beat-up furniture. His examination room is a curtained-off closet that barely holds two chairs. The beds, all filled, are stashed in corridors and corners. The whole place is in desperate need of a decent coat of paint. "Everyone in this field burns out sooner or later, and they burn out multiple times before they quit," Dr. Zeit says. "There are only so many times you can come in at night and see fifty people waiting."

Over the past couple of years, I've written many columns in the *Globe and Mail* about Canada's deteriorating health care system. Nothing has struck me more forcefully than the toll it's taking on its professionals — the nurses, doctors, and hospital administrators who are trying to keep it stuck together with chewing gum and bailing wire. They will say what the politicians will not: The status quo cannot be sustained.

The people on the front lines of medicine are dedicated professionals who are immensely frustrated by a system that no longer works. They're burned out and fed up. Their collected voices say more than stacks of policy papers ever can: The time for fundamental change is here.

It's Hard to be a Baby Doctor

Keith MacLeod is part of a dying breed. He works ninety hours a week. He once delivered 800 babies in a single year. But no one wants to work those hours any more, or be on call around the clock, or train ten years for a profession whose rewards are increasingly modest.

Dr. MacLeod practises in Windsor, which has ten obstetricians to deliver 4,500 babies a year. Across the border, in Detroit, an obstetrician's average caseload is 180 babies a year. "If we had our volumes and their fees," he says, "we'd all be as rich as Bill Gates." So far, the province hasn't capped the number of babies it allows to be born. But Dr. MacLeod makes less money per birth than a midwife. He gets $333 ($70 extra for a C-section).

Family doctors can deliver babies too, but few of them do. It doesn't make financial sense for them because their insurance premiums would soar. And many family doctors are now women with their own families. They don't want the crazy hours that bringing babies into the world entails.

One-third of Canada's obstetricians will retire over the next decade or so. But obstetrics is such an undesirable line of work that medical schools can't find enough people to fill the sixty spots available for obstetricians-in-training. And once they graduate, up to one-third of our new obstetricians head straight for the United States. It's not just the money or the taxes — it's the chance to practise medicine and also have a reasonable life.

Why Small-Town Doctors Want to Quit

Mary Ann Bramstrup is a family doctor with two offices in New Brunswick: one in Fredericton, and one in a smaller town nearby. "An old country doctor, that's what I am," she says (in fact, she's only forty-five). In spring 2000 she decided she was burning out, so she put the Fredericton half of her practice on the market — for free. "The market down here is so poor, the value of medical practices is zero."

The problem is not lack of patients, but too many of them. New Brunswick has fewer physicians than almost anywhere in the country, and every one of them is swamped. "I'm working harder than I did ten years ago for less money," she says. "I can't keep caught up."

And what will happen to her patients if Dr. Bramstrup gets no offers? "They'll just scatter. The other doctors won't take them."

New Brunswick's Physician Resource Allocation Plan is a good example of how not to solve doctor shortages. The plan bribes young, debt-laden docs to move to rural areas, work hard, and pay off their medical school loans. But if they want to move to the city a few years later, the province takes away their billing number. The end result? New doctors won't take the deal. Or if they do, they'll move to Nova Scotia or Ontario or North Carolina before long.

At the other end of the country, Margaret McDiarmid practises medicine in Trail, BC. "I have to personally lobby every day to get what my patients should just automatically get," she admits. "I see a patient, feel a lump. She's fifty-five. Is it ovarian cancer? I have to lobby to get the test done, lobby to get her a quick appointment with the gynecologist. Then the gynecologist has to lobby to get the surgery done. You're constantly apologizing to your patients for what you can't do."

Dr. McDiarmid, who's forty-three, had never been politically involved until now. Like other rural doctors across the province, she threatened to go on strike in the fall of 1999 over low pay and awful working conditions.

Dr. McDiarmid's own father died in 1999 at a hospital in Victoria. The nurses were harassed and overworked, and the nursing care he got was poor. "I was never in favour of privatized medicine before," she says. "But I would have done anything to get good care for my dad."

The Young Nurse

Christine Peterson is a surgical nurse at the Royal Alexandra Hospital in Edmonton. She's in the float pool and carries a pager so the hospital can find her to fill in on short notice. As a casual worker she has no fixed hours, no benefits, and no job security. She works nights, weekends — whenever.

She works twelve-hour shifts that stretch into thirteen. "You don't make a lot of plans," she laughs.

At twenty-five, Christine has been a nurse for only three years and says she's "not militant in the least." But she did support the nurses' plan to strike in Alberta, even illegally if necessary. "The nurses I work with feel they are owed," she says.

So do nurses all across the country. When health care money dried up in the mid-1990s, nursing jobs got chopped just as the pressures on nurses increased. The patients today are sicker and pass through the hospital quicker. Schedules are tight and bed usage is managed down to the minute. There's no time for human interaction. Nurses say it doesn't feel like nursing any more — it feels like an assembly line.

All hospitals today rely on casual workers like Christine. Many nurses have to patch together a living from part-time jobs at different hospitals. The combination of layoffs and rigid union rules has created a nightmare for hospital administrators and nurses alike. Every time someone leaves, there's a chain of consequences that has people moving from one work unit to another. Nurses have been bounced around from job to job, forced to pick up new skills without any extra pay. But promotion and mobility are heavily governed by seniority rather than ability and skills. And the unions have taken away so much flexibility, especially in smaller hospitals, that some good nurses' skills are wasted.

Nurses earn less than teachers and work worse hours. Perhaps the only advantage they have over teachers is their overwhelming popularity with the general public, who in survey after survey, agree that nurses are underpaid and overworked.

Christine always wanted to be a nurse, and she's a good one. But she's not sure she'll be able to stick it out. "Some days I come home after a lot of heavy work, and I'm too tired to talk to my husband," she says. "If I'd known I'd have to work this hard, I honestly don't know if I would have chosen this career."

Nurses: A Great Canadian Export

Fourteen years ago, nurse Linda Beechinor left Canada and moved to Hawaii. She's never looked back. Today, she makes an excellent living recruiting other Canadian nurses to work there. Not only is Hawaii union-friendly, but it has a low nurse-to-patient ratio, great weather, and lots and lots of beaches. "The working conditions are just great here!" she enthuses. "There are plenty of full-time jobs with full benefits, and the base salary is U.S.$50,000."

Canadian nurses have a splendid reputation in the U.S. "Nursing education in Canada is excellent," says Ms. Beechinor. "Too bad the health care system doesn't follow through. You taxpayers are really selling yourselves short."

Plenty of her recruits come from Quebec. One of them, at twenty-seven, landed a secure and highly specialized job as a bone marrow transplant nurse. Back home she would be working gruelling casual shifts, with no benefits, for $35,000 or less. In Hawaii she makes U.S.$55,000.

Ms. Beechinor figures she's brought more than 400 Canadian nurses to Hawaii. "We always have a big party on Canada Day," she says. "We all go to the beach and fly the Maple Leaf."

The Joys of Opting Out

There's no doctor shortage in laser eye surgery. No lineups, either. Laser eye clinics are cheery places where everyone's happy and client service is outstanding. On your way out the door you get a free t-shirt and a customer satisfaction survey.

My myopia was fixed by a highly skilled surgeon named Dr. B, who did a fellowship at Harvard and has won lots of awards. He doesn't do public medicine any more — he's opted out. And who can blame him?

If Dr. B were removing cataracts, the government would regulate his every move. He'd be on quota. The government would tell him how many, at what price, and when demand exceeds supply . . . too bad.

In the private sector there's no imbalance between supply and demand. The waiting time for laser surgery is two weeks and the price has been driven way down by competition. But if you're going blind from cataracts, the waiting time for surgery is up to a year and a half. There are exceptions, of course. If you're American, you can come up to Canada and pay to have your cataracts removed right away by the very same eye surgeons who operate on Canadians. If you're a dog you don't have to wait, either.

Dr. B loves his work. "It's wonderful to treat happy, satisfied patients," he told me. He doesn't have to plead with a hospital board for funds to buy the latest piece of equipment, or ask government bureaucrats where he's allowed to establish his practice. He sets his own hours and gets to go cycling with his kids on weekends.

Dr. B's a happy doctor. It's no surprise he's opted out; it's amazing that more doctors have not.

How We Punish the Specialists

For Martha Hoyt and Joan Murphy, the health care crisis is an intensely personal struggle. Martha Hoyt has survived two bouts of ovarian cancer. Joan Murphy is her doctor.

Ovarian cancer is a deadly disease. Each year 2,500 women in Canada receive this dreadful diagnosis, and fewer than half of them make it to the five-year mark. "I'm one of the lucky ones," says Martha Hoyt.

But Ms. Hoyt might lose her doctor soon. Dr. Murphy is exhausted and fed up with a system so perverse that it punishes our most highly trained physicians. "I really like what I do," she says. "But I will not have my own children pay for the inequities in the system."

Dr. Murphy treats the sickest people of all — those who, like Martha Hoyt, require complex procedures and intensive follow-up. She trained for eleven years to become a gynecological oncologist and is one of only sixteen of these specialists in the province. But she's paid by a piecework system, also known as fee-for-service. One fee fits all, and that means she makes less money than the doctors who refer their toughest cases to her. Over the past decade, cancer doctors' incomes have been driven down and their workload has been driven up.

Three of the other people in Dr. Murphy's subspecialty are weighing offers from the United States. In Ontario, only two new doctors in the past nine years have chosen to train in the field. The province needs twenty Joan Murphys to provide a reasonable standard of care.

Martha Hoyt does advocacy work for ovarian cancer survivors. Their most urgent issue, she says, is trying to keep these specialists in the system. "If we lose even one of these doctors, it could mean delays in diagnosis and delays in surgery and possibly treatment," she pleads.

Dr. Murphy gets less than $600 for performing ovarian cancer surgery. She gets $17 for a follow-up visit. Her teaching and research are done for the love of it. After she pays her professional expenses, she makes less than $200,000 a year (cardiac surgeons make $400,000 to $600,000). She has next to no paid pension plan. There's no Caddy, no cottage, no private schools. She is forty-nine, and a comfortable retirement at sixty-five is not in the cards.

Some people might call Dr. Murphy selfish. Others might wonder why in the world she is still practising medicine in a country that treats her with so little regard. Right now she has a job offer from Florida for twice the money and half the taxes, plus free orthodontics for her kids and a generous pension. "I don't want to leave," she says. But she's not sure she can afford not to.

"Joan Murphy is more than my caregiver," says Martha. "We are partners together. If I lose her, it would be devastating."

How to Jump the Queue

Dr. Arnold Aberman is an expert on waiting lists. As dean of the University of Toronto's medical school during most of the 1990s, he also became one of the most popular guys in town. Everyone called him to try to beat the queue. "Three or four times a week, sometimes, I would arrange preferred access to medical care," he says. "I wasn't proud of it, to tell you the truth, because by helping someone I knew, I was hurting someone I didn't know. It's a zero-sum game."

Many of those who asked Dr. Aberman to pull strings were staunch advocates of preserving medicare as we know it. One was a newspaper executive whose paper deplores queue jumping. Others were top bureaucrats and politicians. "I once got a call from an assistant deputy minister who had twisted her ankle," he recalls. "She asked if I could arrange for her to see an orthopedic surgeon immediately." He could. Two weeks later he sat on a panel with her as she delivered the standard glowing defence of the system. She was proud, she said, that in Canada no one can buy his or her way in to see a specialist.

Dr. Aberman chose to say nothing. After all, he confessed, "she controlled the money for our medical school." The staunchest defenders of the status quo, he observes, include plenty of people who don't have to put up with it.

How We Guaranteed a Doctor Shortage

Dr. Mo Watanabe, the former dean of the University of Calgary's medical school, is Canada's leading expert on the doctor shortage. Ten years ago, he informed me, the bureaucrats allowed 1,753 people a year into Canadian medical schools. In 1997, they allowed 1,415 to enter. Now they've opened the doors a bit wider, but not wide enough to avert a doctor shortage that will plague us for at least another decade.

The health care bureaucrats didn't count on this scenario. Ten years ago they were wringing their hands over the prospect of too many doctors, not too few. Too many doctors would cost too much. Conveniently, the most influential health care economists of the day assured them that cutting back on doctors would actually improve the system.

Then the provinces imposed various other restrictions on the greedy doctors. They capped incomes. They penalized new doctors for settling in cities, hoping this would persuade them to settle in doctor-starved rural areas instead. And they cut back hospital facilities so far that many specialists can now only do surgery one or two days a week.

Plenty of doctors responded to these incentives by leaving the country. In the past decade, more than 4,000 of them have gone. "I don't think anyone anticipated that many of the young physicians would leave the way they did," says Dr. Watanabe. "Nobody took them seriously when they said they'd leave." The doctors tell him they didn't leave because of the money. They left because the U.S. welcomed them with open arms. "In Canada, they just got tired of feeling, day in and day out, that they were the problem."

Because it takes so long to train a doctor, the cutbacks of the early 1990s are only now beginning to be felt. Dr. Watanabe warns that the worst may be yet to come.

The Perfect Storm

At the beginning of September 2000, Dr. Richard Finley did surgery to improve the condition of a patient with severe asthma. She'd originally been scheduled for March 1999. Time and again she was bumped by cases more urgent than hers: gunshot wounds, heart bypasses — the life-threatening rather than the life-impairing.

Dr. Finley is the chief surgeon at Vancouver General, one of Canada's largest hospitals. "I call this 'the perfect storm,'" he told me. "We're out there in the storm with our patients, and there's no help in sight." At the time of our conversation, the hospital's surgeons were threatening a job action.

Canada has never been so rich. But at Vancouver General, the operating rooms function only four days a week. A surgeon gets one day a week in the OR. Surgeries were down more than 10 percent from the year before and were scheduled to fall even further. The reason? Budget cutbacks, and a desperate nursing shortage. Conditions have gotten so bad that surgeons won't take jobs there. "We've tried to hire eight surgeons in the last two years, and all have turned us down," Dr. Finley says.

Shortly after our conversation, the federal government unlocked several billion dollars in health care funding. But Dr. Finley believes there's no quick fix for nearly a decade of cutbacks and bad planning. "These are going to prove to be very expensive policy mistakes," he said.

Anyone Care to Chip In for an MRI?

Tino Martinez is a horse doctor in Victoria. He has a portable ultrasound unit that he uses to diagnose his patients' pregnancies or lameness. So when the local hospital offered him an old ultrasound unit for free, he was delighted. But when he turned it on, all he got was a fuzzy blur. "I thought I was doing something wrong," he says. The unit was simply so old that it was useless. He turned it down, and the hospital tried to donate it to the Third World. But the Third World turned it down, too.

Many hospital back rooms are medical museums of obsolete technology where highly trained radiologists do their best to diagnose your brain tumour, your breast cancer, or your blocked artery with equipment that scarcely works.

One leading Ottawa hospital made do until recently with an angiography machine that was twenty-five years old. (These machines show pictures of your blood vessels, so doctors can decide if you need a heart bypass.) It was so decrepit that it would jam midway through a test, and the anesthetized patient would have to be rolled aside while the technicians got it going again. "In most hospitals, it's almost impossible to replace equipment until it dies," says Ian Hammond, the Ottawa radiologist who told me this story. "It's crisis management. Most hospitals are running deficits, and one piece of expensive X-ray equipment might cost you a million dollars. So do you buy that? Or do you buy incubators instead?"

In Saskatoon, one hospital's angiography machine broke down forty-five times in six months, and the ultrasound unit had to be shut off because it was useless. The radiologists figured their urgent new equipment needs would cost $14 million. When the big squeeze came on hospital budgets, they stopped spending on equipment. Many major hospitals haven't had a capital replacement budget for a decade. We're paying the price now. More than half of Canada's X-ray, ultrasound, and other imaging equipment has outlived its useful life.

At the same time, rapid technological advances have put expensive tools such as CT scanners and MRIs at the heart of good patient care. "When I started in medicine, if nobody knew what was wrong with you, we cut you open and looked inside," says Dr. Hammond. "This equipment has revolutionized medicine." Demand for MRIs is so heavy that even some private MRI clinics have waiting lists.

Canada's stock of medical equipment is way behind most of Europe's. It's worse than Hungary's or the Czech Republic's. "In Europe," says one expert, "there would be a total revolt of the medical community."

The federal government has promised a billion dollars for new X-ray machines, MRIs, and CT scanners. But we probably need two or three times that much to catch up. And that's why, in many parts of Canada today, a horse can get a better scan than a person can.

Health Care Hypocrisy and MRIs

At the end of 1999 a flap broke out in Ontario when some MRI clinics were caught accepting payments directly from patients who didn't want to wait eight months or more in line. Judging by the outrage, you'd think these clinics were drowning puppies. "It is illegal to have anyone pay for medically necessary services," pronounced Ontario's health minister. The *Toronto Star* opined that treatments for cash threaten the very foundation of medicare.

But what's illegal in Ontario is perfectly legal in Alberta, British Columbia, and Quebec, where private MRI clinics are flourishing. Even Ontario has a two-tier MRI payment system, with preferred access for some. The Toronto Blue Jays and the Toronto Raptors have (perfectly legal) hospital contracts for their players, who are seen right away. The Workers' Compensation Board also pays for speedy MRIs for injured workers. Private insurers and lawyers pay for people injured in motor vehicle accidents and other clients with personal injury cases. Such third party business has become an important source of revenue for cash-starved hospitals.

Magnetic resonance imaging supplies an excellent example of how our inflexible, bureaucratic monster of a medical system has sentenced us to second-rate health care. MRI technology has been around for less than twenty years. It's been called the best diagnostic tool on the planet, far more effective than X-rays or CT scans, and it has changed the way medicine is done. "I can't tell you how beautiful it is," says Rosemary Haeckel, an MRI technician who works at a private clinic in Edmonton. "It gives you amazing pictures of soft tissue. You can see all the bones, ligaments, and muscles. The only way to get better pictures is to take a really sharp knife and cut your body in half."

Doctors keep finding more things that MRIs can do, and demand for the scans has exploded. In Alberta, for example, MRI use has tripled in five years. But the supply of machines hasn't kept up. They are expensive — $3 million or more to buy the machine and build a clinic — and until recently, governments didn't fund them. Canada has fewer MRIs per capita than Iceland, Hungary, South Korea, and the Czech Republic.

MRI scanning is a good candidate for private enterprise because it can be done efficiently in stand-alone clinics. Meadowlark MRI in Edmonton, where Rosemary Haeckel works, is a business venture by a group of entrepreneurial radiologists. Meadowlark competes with other private operators and bills at a rate much cheaper than the under-the-table private fees charged in Ontario.

But the very idea of competition makes health care bureaucrats and *Toronto Star* editorial writers break out in hives. It also makes them break out in high-minded rhetoric designed to defend a system of equal and fair access that exists only in their imaginations.

The Radiologists

Ila Branscombe was a young university student in Regina when she was diagnosed with terminal brain cancer. Surgery was useless, she was told. Only radiation therapy might prolong her life. So Ila's brain was bombarded with radiation. She had to take powerful steroids. Her hair fell out. She gained ninety pounds and began to suffer memory loss. A few months later, she learned the tumour was still growing and she had only a few months to live.

Then she sought a second opinion. It turned out that the original pathologist's diagnosis was wrong and she didn't have cancer after all. But it was too late. The devastating treatment left her with permanent brain damage. Once, she'd planned to be a designer. Now she collects a disability pension.

In any health care system, medical mistakes and misdiagnoses are un-avoidable. But Canada's diagnostic specialists have become so overloaded that their operations are a breeding ground for error. That's the message from some of the country's top pathologists — the doctors who read your breast biopsy or your Pap smear and figure out what type of treatment might be best. In Canada, they diagnose 600,000 patients a year.

In January 2000, seven of Canada's leading pathologists appeared on the television documentary program *W Five*. "We've been silent for too long," said one. "I [will not be able to] stand behind the quality of work that is going to come out of my laboratory," said another. The group included Diponkar Bannerjee, chief of hematopathology at Toronto's Princess Margaret Hospital, the leading cancer care facility in Canada. Another doctor who appeared was Patricia Shaw, a gynecological pathologist at Toronto's Sunnybrook Hospital. She's a key part of the cancer team there. "Our workloads have gone up arguably as much as 70 percent at Sunnybrook," she said. "It's gotten out of control."

This country currently has only two-thirds the number of pathologists recommended for our population base. We need thirty to fifty new ones each year just to replace the people who are retiring. But in 2000, only ten new pathologists started training.

Pathologists are employed by hospitals and the evisceration of hospital budgets has hit them hard. Across Canada, they complain about administrators oblivious to their needs and vanishing support staff. But it's hard to pin the blame on the administrators, who are trying to manage shortages all over.

Dr. Shaw spends her days looking through a microscope, concentrating on tiny pieces of tissue. What she does is part science and part art. "If we get tired, we start to slip up," she confesses. "Sometimes you know you should show it [the sample] around for a second opinion, but you tend to cut corners." No matter how fast and accurately they work, pathologists all agree that delays in diagnosis are a mounting medical problem.

In the meantime, the shortage has become so acute that in some areas, doctors are allowed to do this specialty work even if they've flunked their pathology exams several times over. The worst shortage in the country is in Ila Branscombe's province, Saskatchewan.

Traumatized by Health Care Politics

Early one morning in September 2000, Christian Yau was riding his motor-cycle to work when he hit a rut in the road. The next thing he remembers is being in an ambulance heading to the nearest hospital. The ER doctors tested him from head to foot and found a broken pelvis, a broken wrist, bruised lungs, and a severely lacerated liver. And that's when his troubles really began.

His bleeding liver was life-threatening, and he needed to be transferred to a trauma hospital quickly; the next hour or two would be critical. But not a single trauma centre in Greater Vancouver had room for him. The thirty-one-year-old aircraft mechanic waited for twelve hours in the ER as doctors watched his vital signs and frantically phoned for help. At long last, he was put on a helicopter to the Harborview hospital in Seattle. "The ER doctors had to go through a lot of hoops and red tape to get permission," he told me.

Harborview is a regional trauma centre that serves five states and treats all comers, regardless of where they're from or whether they can pay. "At Harborview," Mr. Yau says, "they don't say no to anybody."

A couple of weeks after his accident, doctors at Vancouver General, the province's leading hospital, went public to warn that other accident victims are dying because of delays in treatment. Some politicians accused the doctors of playing health care politics. Mr. Yau knew otherwise. "We're just going nuts here," admits Richard Simons, head of the trauma care pro-gram. "We're here to take care of patients and we just can't do it because we can't get them in here."

And that's not the hospital's only problem. It's also a victim of a deeply politicized health care administration. In the midst of the trauma crisis, the hospital's president and its entire board of trustees were fired without warning. The dismissals were directed by David Levi, a long-time NDP operative who also chairs the Vancouver-Richmond Health Board.

Mr. Levi, who was openly dissatisfied with the now ex-president, says the group was fired to streamline administration and save money. Insiders say it was a politically motivated power grab inspired, in part, by union oppo-sition over the hospital's plan to build a (nonunion) biotechnology park.

British Columbia's health board wields tremendous power. But few of its members know much about health care. They are nearly all outsiders. Insiders, the thinking went, would make the board too biased in favour of

doctors, nurses, and hospitals. So British Columbia's health care policy —
as well as its most important teaching, research, and treatment centre — is
in the hands of people who know very little about hospitals or medicine.

The doctors' relationship with Mr. Levi's health board has been terrible.
The acting president of the medical staff, John Wade, said that dismissing
the hospital's "sensational" volunteer board in the midst of the trauma crisis was like "firing the surgeon in the middle of an operation and asking a
medical school student to finish." As one aghast insider puts it, "This is a
hospital run amok."

Chaos at Hamilton's Superhospital

The meltdown at Canada's biggest superhospital in spring 2000 barely
registered as a media story. Perhaps that's because the facility is located in
Hamilton, just down the road from Toronto, and no national journalist
lives there.

Hamilton's superhospital is made up of several different hospitals,
uneasily merged. The Hamilton Health Sciences Corporation, as it's called,
serves two million people in booming Southern Ontario. The HHSC has a
budget of half a billion dollars a year and employs 8,000 people. In medical and teaching expertise, it's among the jewels of the system.

And it hit the wall. Among its problems is a deficit heading toward
$90 million and a desperate doctor shortage. William Shragge, the HHSC's
chief of medical staff, says, "I've got doctors crashing, working thirty and
forty hours straight because there aren't enough of them. If the status quo
is maintained, programs will crash, and waiting times for some surgery
will triple." ER doctor Dennis Psutka notes, "Our emergency rooms have
been turned into wards. Almost all those people are waiting for beds. So
now, when I see new people at emergency, I see them in chairs or in a
closet."

Dr. Shragge describes a lopsided seller's market for doctors. "Many physicians here have three or four offers on the table," he said. "We brought a
recruit in recently, a young internist. He spent two weeks here and left. He
said the working conditions are intolerable."

The superhospital's problems have many tangled roots. But the over-
reaching problem is (as always) money. There weren't enough dollars in
the budget (set by the province) to keep all the sites and programs going.
The board of trustees had proposed a plan, but consultants hired by

Ontario's Health Ministry didn't like it. The consultants issued a damning report that blasted the administration and also condemned the trustees for putting patient care ahead of fiscal responsibility.

Ontario's health minister responded by firing the trustees and the chief administrator. She put the HHSC under provincial supervision, and appointed an all-powerful supervisor to clean up the mess. Soon after that, she admitted that the hospital could not get by on its budget, and increased its funding by the same amount the trustees had asked for in the first place.

Hamilton was supposed to reap efficiencies from the province's exercise in hospital restructuring. But as it turned out, restructuring cost much more than anyone expected and the province wound up having to restore much of the money and many of the beds it had taken out of the system. But bricks and mortar and beds represent the easy part — finding the human resources to care for sick people will be far more difficult.

At Last, a Happy Patient

Sandra Hughes is a big fan of Canadian health care. As a long-time patient of the Vancouver Breast Centre, she has nothing but the highest praise for the treatment she gets there, especially after she was diagnosed with a tiny precancerous lump in her breast a few months ago.

Sandra could write an ad for the place. The headline would read "Patients Come First." Her mammograms are personally supervised by Linda Warren, an international expert in diagnostic imaging. Then Dr. Warren herself shows Sandra the X-ray and explains it in plain language. Sandra doesn't have to wait and worry for weeks. She gets the results the same day. "My surgeon said if Warren hadn't circled my cancer on the mammogram, he wouldn't have seen it," Sandra informs me. "That's how good she is."

So what's the catch? Sandra's an American who comes here for health care. Because she's a paying customer, she's allowed to skip the lines and the hassles in order to purchase first-rate doctoring.

Canadians cannot get what Sandra gets.

Our system doesn't pay Dr. Warren anywhere enough for that. The fee schedule pays her just $73.66 to read your X-ray. After expenses, she nets around $8.

That's one reason why there's a shortage of radiologists.

The breast centre where Dr. Warren works delivers two-tier service. One tier provides the government-funded, stripped-down, assembly-line version of care. The other tier provides the kind of care that Sandra gets and it attracts women from all around the world, as well as new Canadians who aren't covered by health insurance.

Some of these women are rich, but many are not. Sandra Hughes, sixty-five, is a travel writer who lives in Bellingham, WA. "I buy bread on sale!" she laughs. At $185 per visit, she thinks the breast centre is a bargain.

Now the Vancouver Breast Centre has quietly begun to offer its premium service to Canadians. "As doctors, we're very concerned about the level of care we can deliver to patients," says Ian Gardiner, one of the doctors who founded the facility. "It's really boosted morale because here we can deliver quality care and not be dictated to by some health care bureaucrat."

Because people pay realistic fees, the breast centre can afford all sorts of market-sensitive amenities that the public system deems "not medically necessary." It has a multilingual staff and a reference library. The appointments last at least half an hour. Most importantly, it can organize itself around the needs of its patients. "In the public system it's up to you to be an advocate for your own health," says Gardiner. "Sure, the family doctor will help, but he's very busy."

Is this the tip of the iceberg? "Absolutely no question about it." Dr. Gardiner continues, "Canadians want something more than what the government will provide. Eventually, the public is just going to demand the kind of service they want, and the politicians will have to explain to them why they can't have it."

Some of Canada's best physicians are opting partway or all the way out of the system so they can practise more satisfying medicine. Opting out frees them from the assembly-line medicine that's burning out so many doctors. It also allows them to make more money. So long as governments think that reading a patient's mammogram is worth eight bucks, it's hard to blame them.

Our public system can't afford the kind of personal care that Sandra gets. Is it immoral to allow people the choice of paying extra if they want it? Sandra doesn't think so. She thinks the question is a little nutty.

SECOND THOUGHTS

William Orovan

For many medicare apologists, health care problems are transient or, worse, merely created by those with vested interests in the system (e.g., physicians) to extract new health care dollars. It's a heavy charge, but most Canadian physicians have remained quiet on the issue. Dr. William Orovan, however, made national news in 1998 when, as president of the Ontario Medical Association (OMA), he addressed the Empire Club. In his speech, Orovan not only questioned the quality of care, but went even further: he challenged the purpose of the Canada Health Act and the structural problems the legislation has created.

In this interview, Orovan discusses his views on medicare and his reasons for joining in the public — and often bitter — debate over health care reform. "I have children. I live in this province. I'm a citizen of this country, in addition to being a practising physician. I want to be sure that every citizen has available to him or her quality, timely health care when he or she needs it. I'm convinced that if we carry on as we are now, we're in for some very serious trouble. I can't sit back and just allow this to happen." Orovan's commitment is remarkable given that he did his fellowship training at the MD Anderson Cancer Center in Houston, TX, where he was offered a position. Instead, he chose to come home.

Orovan, a practising surgeon who has served in a variety of administrative positions, is unequivocal in his evaluation of the system: "We have major, major issues, and I don't think 'crisis' is too strong a term to apply to this situation. We're fortunate in that we have a little bit of lead time here before the real crunch . . ."

He expresses disappointment with the current trend toward the bureaucratization of health care in the name of reform. "Doctors ought to use their time for what they're trained to do: deliver care. More and more of their time is being consumed by trying to deal with the system, whether it's prescribing drugs or getting a test scheduled or arranging home care."

Describing the Canada Health Act as a straightjacket, Orovan observes, "Nobody would suggest that the way we did things thirty years ago in any other area of endeavour should be the way we do things today. We made one adjustment to the Canada Health Act about seventeen years ago when we introduced the fifth principle, that of 'accessibility.' Since 1968, we have not had a serious reexamination of the principles. We have this introspective, almost ostrich-like approach to it: stick our heads in the sand and convince ourselves that this is the Canadian way."

Dismissing the Fyke report — and similar reform suggestions — as reflecting a "central planning approach," Orovan calls for a new analysis of our health care system, beginning with a debate on the Canada Health Act. Drawing on international examples, he advocates a greater role for private financing and delivery of services.

I joined Dr. Orovan in the offices of the Ontario Medical Association in May 2000. [**DG** = Dr. David Gratzer; **WO** = Dr. William Orovan]

DG: There are roughly 55,000 physicians in this country. Most never write a letter to the editor. Why have you chosen to get involved in the health care debate?

WO: Health care is one of the most important social programs in Canada. I don't subscribe to the idea that medicare is what distinguishes us as Canadians, but the future of health care is important to all Canadians. I have children. I live in this province. I'm a citizen of this country, in addition to being a practising physician. I want to be sure that every citizen has available to him or her quality, timely health care when he or she needs it. I'm convinced that if we carry on as we are now, we're in for some very serious trouble. I can't sit back and just allow this to happen.

DG: The health care debate in Canada is so terribly controversial and fraught with emotion. Even the question of whether or not there is a problem with the standards of care today is controversial. In the fall, CBC Radio did a forum and they titled it *Crisis, What Crisis?* Bob Evans, a British Columbia health economist, suggested several months ago in an international journal that confidence in Canada's health care system is low because of Conrad

Black and his newspapers, and if we had more accurate reporting, people would not feel that way. As a practising physician, what do you make of that argument?

WO: It's absolute nonsense. The only people who could ever say that there's no problem in health care today in Canada are those who are distant from the system, or have no direct contact with the system. For the doctors and the nurses and the other health care professionals who are practising on a daily basis, it's obvious that there are serious problems, not just with the quality of care, but with the morale of those who are delivering it.

Doctors are leaving Canada in large numbers. I grant you some are coming back, but there's a significant net loss every year. Nurses are leaving the country — or are leaving the profession — in droves and waiting lists are getting longer. I know that it's difficult to quantify that because the data available is not good.

I think we can say that in spite of all the difficulties, we've still managed to maintain a reasonable level of quality of care. When you do get to the front of the line, the care that you get is pretty darn good. I think that's because of the dedicated professionals who deliver it, many of whom are aging and thinking of retirement. We are, in addition to that, dependent now on a significant number of doctors who are working beyond retirement age. When they retire, the impact on waiting lists will be very significant.

But to say that there's not a crisis now, and indeed to suggest that some-how things are going to be just fine if we don't do something, is totally disingenuous. As you know, there is the issue of aging and the changing demographics in the population, and the tremendous impact that technology is going to have. In many industries, technology has resulted in the lowering of costs, but that virtually has never happened in medicine.

We have major, major issues, and I don't think "crisis" is too strong a term to apply to this situation. We're fortunate in that we have a little bit of lead time here before the real crunch, when the baby boomers start to get into their seventh decade and really make demands on the health care sys-tem. And I think you can't be too emphatic about the fact that we need a vigorous debate. We need a plan of action. We need it now, or this system is going to founder.

DG: You make a very forceful argument, but when you're in debate, often you're challenged on those basic assumptions. Take the waiting list issue. You recently participated in a television panel discussion on *Michael Coren*

Live. You brought up waiting lists and Carol Kushner, a health consultant and author, immediately said that the waiting list data is unreliable and that you're fear-mongering. How do you respond to that?

WO: Well, she's right that the data is not complete. We have private practitioners delivering the care in most circumstances and, for hospital-based care, we don't keep good statistics. In general, operating room waiting times, for instance, are not known because we don't require that surgeons put in their list until seven days in advance.

The evidence we *do* have, however, suggests there is a very major problem in diagnostic imaging and numerous interventional procedures. In my own hospital, we've seen a twofold increase in the CT scan waiting list over the last three years, even though we've added machine capacity. And, with regard to MRIs, we're slowly getting the waiting list down to something that might be considered nearly acceptable by the dramatic addition of twenty-eight new MRI machines in the province of Ontario in the last eighteen months.

Data is also available for cataract extraction; we know there are huge waiting lists. I get calls frequently from people saying, "My mother's seventy-five years old, she has a cataract and can't read. She likes to watch television and she can't." Cataracts have a big impact on quality of life for these people who have limited life expectancy and face long waiting times.

I know these are anecdotes. Anecdotes aren't evidence — we need to generate better data on waiting lists. But it's not fear-mongering to tell the truth.

DG: You're also a practising surgeon, specializing in oncological cases. Have you seen examples from your own practice where patients have waited longer than clinically ideal?

WO: Absolutely. A colleague — who is a full-time practising surgical oncologist — calls me regularly to say that he has people with invasive bladder cancer and there's no opportunity to get them to the operating room for three, four, five months. In some cases I've been able to help out, but treatment waiting times are too long.

I know that many surgical oncologists in the community — who are in full-time practice — are finding it extraordinarily difficult to get operating room time or radiation oncology services. Radiation oncology, particularly for prostate cancer and breast cancer, is another area where the waiting lists are well documented.

So there are some examples of waiting lists that are excessive. We are compromising care and increasing the risk to patients — not just risk of advancing disease, but there's a serious psychological issue as well, for instance, for women with breast cancer. The psychological impact of long waiting times is huge.

DG: You have a unique perspective. You're not just a practising surgeon — you also have had many other roles to play. Within the Ontario Medical Association [OMA], you were the chief negotiator. You have been the acting dean of a university faculty. You've served in the senior administration of a hospital. In those different roles, have you seen the stress on the health care system?

WO: I have been fortunate to have had many roles within health care delivery and within the physician community, and I can reinforce that there are extreme levels of stress on all providers, physicians, nurses, and support workers. All of them are burdened by the issues involved in providing quality clinical care and are exhausted by the requirements put on them on a day-to-day basis. They have very little left to give.

We've done surveys within the OMA that suggest that 40 percent of doctors are considering retiring within the next five years. Two-thirds of doctors are thinking about — or have thought about in the past five years — emigrating elsewhere, usually to the United States. A significant number — although not as many as in nursing — are thinking of leaving the profession.

And it's always the same thing. It's the incredible burden of work. It's the attempt to try and balance the needs of your patient with the inadequacies of the system and still try to have some kind of a semblance of life for yourself and for your family. I see it among physicians all the time.

DG: Doctors seem very frustrated with the system. That's reflected in polling data commissioned by the OMA, as well as other health associations across the country. There's also the exodus of physicians; it's down marginally from its peak in the mid-1990s, but it's still dramatically higher than anything we saw through the 1980s and in the early 1990s. And yet, there seems to be such a reluctance on the part of providers in general, and physicians in particular, to get involved in the health care debate. Even medical associations seem generally hesitant to wade in. I think your comments, and your successor's comments, are pretty unique in terms of criticizing the system. Why aren't physicians more active and involved?

WO: Physicians, like other members of society, recognize that there is a significant need for change. Physicians have supported this view through their respective associations, but there remains a lot of uncertainty about how we should change the system and what change will mean for individual providers and for patients.

As well, this debate has become so politicized and so emotional that there's reluctance to make your feelings known because of the vituperative nature of the replies. We're into questioning people's motives rather than examining their ideas. It's a harsh environment. Physicians — while they definitely want what's best for their patients — are reluctant to be labelled or to have their motives questioned. It's not unusual or unexpected to see people shy away from that.

DG: The Harvard School of Public Health recently did an international study looking at health care in five nations. One area of study: how doctors feel about their system. When asked about the quality of care over the last five years, 59 percent of Canadian family doctors felt that it had worsened. Specialists in Canada were even more negative: some 67 percent hold that same opinion. These are higher percentages of dissatisfaction than in any of the other four nations.

Why are Canadian doctors so much more critical than their colleagues? Changes take place in Australia and the United States. Why are our doctors more negative than doctors from those regions?

WO: The process of change is worldwide and the debate on health care is active in many countries.

In Canada, physicians perceive a significant amount of rigidity within the system. There is very little flexibility, there is inadequate funding, and there is a sense that there are no options or choices available other than trying to prop up what seems to them a failing system.

When you have choices, your level of frustration is reduced. When you perceive that there are no choices — that you're trapped in a system you believe to be inadequate in many respects — then the level of frustration is much higher. It almost seems sometimes that the system is set up to frustrate the needs of physicians and patients, rather than to meet them. The increasing bureaucracy within the system worsens the situation.

The drug benefit formulary in Ontario is a good example. When the use of a specific drug goes up, the system's answer is to impose additional bureaucratic barriers to prescribing that medication. Ciprofloxacin [an antibiotic], for instance, is now on the "limited use" formulary in Ontario, using an argument about increased emergence of organism resistance. The evidence suggests that this is mainly a veterinary phenomenon, rather than a human one. Now, in order to get patients Ciprofloxacin, doctors must fill out a limited use form, which is very time consuming.

It's a counterproductive measure. Doctors ought to use their time for what they're trained to do: deliver care. More and more of their time is being consumed by trying to deal with the system and trying to make the system work for their patients, which involves endless attempts to organize diagnostic testing, to schedule appointments with other busy practitioners or laboratories, and to arrange appropriate treatment. There is an endless series of bureaucratic barriers to providing care.

These problems are not limited to Canada. Dealing with the insurance companies in the United States must be at least as frustrating. There are, however, other systems, particularly in other OECD [Organisation for Economic Co-Operation and Development] countries, where solutions have been found to some of these problems or at least alternative ways of dealing with these extensive nonmedical tasks have been addressed. I think we should look at some of these other alternatives and see what might be possible here in Canada.

DG: You speak from an Ontario perspective, but really these problems apply across the country. There are bureaucratic hurdles to getting home care, drugs, and diagnostic tests. In some way, isn't that the way governments across the country have reformed health care?

WO: Or *not* reformed it!

You're right that there are problems with accessibility across the country. It's hard to have a price/demand curve when there's no price, so demand exceeds the dollars available in every jurisdiction. The tendency on the part of government has been to look to the access point [the physician] and try to find ways of constraining his or her freedoms to act.

DG: Speaking of another country, you have had the opportunity to work in the United States. You worked at the MD Anderson Center in Houston. How was that experience compared with what you see here?

WO: The MD Anderson is part of the University of Texas, which is a publicly funded cancer care network in that state. I have not practised privately in the

United States, and have not seen the kind of difficulties that practitioners and patients face there on a regular basis.

The United States is a fascinating place. The tension and ambition drives the country in a search for excellence. But there are also consequences that aren't at all good. The fact that they have 44 million Americans either uninsured or dramatically underinsured is a huge problem. Accessibility to care for those who can't afford it is a terrible situation that we would never want to allow to happen in Canada.

They've managed to achieve great things as a result of their drive and resources. But American health care is not a system that we should look to as a model. I think we have the will, the knowledge, and — if we're willing to use it — the vision to create a better system in Canada.

DG: The MD Anderson Center is a very unique place to study and practise. The facility has a research budget that's larger than the total amount of money we spend on medical R&D [research and development] in Canada. You were offered a job there. Why did you come back?

WO: Well, I'm Canadian. I have an attachment to this province and this country that goes beyond my profession. My children were born here. My parents were buried here. My family lives here. I want to put my effort into making Canada and making Ontario a better place to live and work and get good health care.

I would have had a very different career in the United States. I might have avoided some of the frustrations and pressures that physicians and patients face in Canada, but I felt that whatever skills I had — clinical and otherwise — I wanted to put them to work in Canada. I have had a good and rewarding clinical practice here for many years. I'm glad I made the decision to come home. I personally have been able to make a minor difference in the way things are done in this country. I was, I think, the first person to do continent urinary diversion in Canada. In the early 1990s, I had the largest series of this procedure in Canada.

I made a small difference clinically, and I hope I can make a further difference in this debate and the future of our health care system.

DG: You speak of coming back to Canada because of your roots and your passion for the country. The harshest attacks you've received for your comments claim that your health care ideas are un-Canadian and what you want is an Americanization of the system. How do you respond?

WO: First of all, such attacks aren't unexpected. The tactic used by those who want the system to remain largely unchanged is to question the motives of those who want to engage in an open debate. I understand the significance that health care and medicare has for Canadians. I respect the spirit of the Canada Health Act, but it has been three decades since the original principles were promulgated and more than fifteen years since any change at all has been made to the provisions of medicare. I think we must revisit these principles.

We simply cannot operate in the twenty-first century without being willing to question every aspect of what we do. We're moving into a global economy. If we're going to remain competitive as a nation, we have to be willing to continue questioning everything we do. And we can't have areas where we say, "Well, it's un-Canadian to question that." It's just anti-intellectual. Humans by nature are outward looking and inquisitive. It's what drives everything we do as a nation — why would health care be any different? Why can we question virtually every other aspect of our political situation, from the monarchy to the Indian Act, but not health care? It's a nonsensical approach. It is, in my view, self-serving on the part of those who, for whatever reason, don't want this discussion to go forward.

Nobody would suggest that the way we did things thirty years ago in any other area of endeavour should be the way we do things today. We made one adjustment to the Canada Health Act about seventeen years ago when we introduced the fifth principle, that of "accessibility." Since 1968, we have had not had a serious reexamination of the principles. We have this introspective, almost ostrich-like approach to it: stick our heads in the sand and convince ourselves that this is the Canadian way.

DG: Why is this such an emotional issue for Canadians? Every other aspect of public policy in Canada is open for discussion. We talk about privatizing the Canada Pension Plan and power generation. We discuss school choice for education. But health care is a different matter. Why is it that the Canada Health Act has become a defining characteristic of our nation?

WO: Why is health important? Obviously, the answer — at least in part — is that it touches everybody in such a significant way. If you do not have good health, then everything else in life becomes problematic. People understand the importance of good health and attach great importance to good health and medical care. Life is good for most people, unlike it was in, say, the Middle Ages, when death seemed to be a respite. Death and disease are things that people desperately want to put off. So health care touches everybody at all ages. For a mother or a child to die in childbirth is virtually unheard of. A hundred years ago, it was common. So people have great expectations. They demand that the health care system be there for them when they need it. And any suggestion, whether by providers or by politicians or by other citizens that this might not be the case, produces a lot of anxiety.

Perhaps this reaction to the concept of change is not so surprising. Change is difficult in virtually every area of endeavour. People — whether in business or in politics — seldom embrace it unless they see no alternative. Maybe we're not quite there yet in health care. When I made my speech to the Empire Club of Canada in November 1998, health care issues were just becoming front-and-centre for Canadians. We never would have believed back then that national media columnists and others would pick up the torch and actually question the Canada Health Act as it now exists.

DG: You touch on the speech. In November 1998 you said, "To begin with, discussion among Canadians about health care is based on the widely held belief that we have the best health care system in the world, but what if that is not true any more? As a matter of fact, I believe it is not true any more."

You went on to "question" the Canada Health Act. Critics have suggested that when you question the Canada Health Act, what you're really suggesting is greater privatization, or a parallel private system. What is it that's wrong with the Canada Health Act, and what ought we do about it?

WO: The Canada Health Act is a straightjacket. It constrains our freedom to act, our ability to look for choices and options, and it doesn't allow us to meet the medical needs of Canadians today.

What does "accessibility" mean? Is it reasonable accessibility to wait six months for an MRI? Is it reasonable accessibility to wait two years for a cataract extraction? Is it reasonable accessibility to wait a year to see an arthroplasty surgeon and another year to have a total joint arthroplasty, which, in terms of improving quality of life, has been shown in several studies to be one of the most effective interventions that we have in medicine?

Another issue is the interpretation of "comprehensive" to include anything that's medically necessary. That term's interpreted across this country in dramatically different ways, depending on whether you're talking about in vitro fertilization or contraception control.

And I don't think that "public administration" is, frankly, something that all Canadians believe in as strongly as some proponents of the Canada Health Act. We have many examples in government policy where services that were once publicly administered are now private. Health care could follow suit. In the last part of the nineteenth century, for example, fire was such a hazard that people strongly advocated — and several jurisdictions had — publicly administered fire insurance. Who, a hundred years later, would suggest that fire insurance is something that ought to be publicly administered? There's been a significant change in that practice.

Thirty years ago, the public administration of health care was felt to be essential. We at least ought to question that view. If the private sector can do it more efficiently, if the private sector can deliver better value for Canadians in health care, why in the world shouldn't we let it?

In terms of a parallel system, I don't have any preordained notions. I do, however, believe in choice and options for providers and patients.

As you look at this whole system, the costs are going to rise. There are several studies by the Conference Board of Canada that suggest in a few short years, given current rates of growth and expected increases in demand, significantly more than 50 percent of all public expenditures by provinces will be devoted to health care. This cost will put at serious risk our other social and infrastructure programs and, quite frankly, we just can't afford it.

So, at the end of the day, if you can't afford a publicly funded system to do everything for everybody, then some choices are necessary. Either you're going to do less and do it for everybody, or you're going to do what you're doing now but do it for fewer people. And frankly, from the point of view of choice, if some people want to de-list themselves voluntarily from the publicly funded system, spend their own resources on health care, and yet continue to support the public system — exactly as we do with public education — I don't see much wrong with that.

DG: With regard to private services, there is an argument that you can actually privatize quite a bit within the present confines of the Canada Health Act. According to Mike Harris, the premier of Ontario, this would be one way of reducing cost. Internationally, that's actually not a controversial idea. The Labour government is running for reelection in Britain with the promise to privatize or transfer to the private sector 200,000 surgeries in the next four years [publicly funded, privately provided]. In Sweden [as described in the essay by Carl Irvine, Johan Hjertqvist, and David Gratzer in this volume], they've privatized everything from home care to ambulance services to the largest hospital in Stockholm, again maintaining public financing. Is this a route you think Canada should go?

WO: I think it's inevitable that we will. There *is* going to be increased cost associated with health care. The question is, how much can we publicly afford, and how much has to be spent or has to be raised or has to be accounted for in other ways? Because costs are going to go up.

Increased private sector funding is absolutely essential. There are many areas in which we can move forward; the traditional areas in which we've had private funding — chronic care, home care, and pharmaceuticals — are not enough. It's with the really expensive parts of health care — acute care, for example — that we're up against this concept: while private spending may be okay for chronic care, home care, and pharmaceuticals, it's un-Canadian to have private spending for acute care.

So it's just not a consistent argument. It's not one that can withstand the kind of rigorous debate that we need to have about health care.

DG: Producing reports on medicare has become a cottage industry in Canada. We have had three provincial reports released within the last three years [in Nova Scotia, Quebec, Saskatchewan]. We have the Senate of Canada working rigorously on a report. And there is the forthcoming Romanow Commission's report. Of the three we already have, probably the most important one was written by Kenneth Fyke for the Saskatchewan Commission on Medicare. It is an influential document due to the rigour of its investigation and its implications for Romanow's final report. Fyke, as you know, worked within the bureaucracy for thirty-five years and was a deputy minister of health.

Fyke's final report — the end product of a year's work — is extraordinarily critical of the health care system. At one point he says that this is a system insensitive to results. At another point he even says that we get a poor return on our dollar, even relative to the American system. And yet at the end of the day, Ken Fyke suggests that we should have — in Saskatchewan, at least — fewer regional health boards, a better annual report, another committee looking at quality standards, and primary care reform. Do you find these suggestions, which are probably going to be replicated in the Romanow report, "in the box"?

WO: Completely. While I recognize all input and dialogue is important, it seems to me that Fyke's is a very leftist philosophy. All we have to do is just manage better, manage more restrictively, and things will be all right. There's a "central planning" approach to his ideas as the preferred solution. That kind of thinking won't move the discussion forward, I'm afraid.

I've spoken on one occasion to Senator Kirby. I had a sense that he was an open, outward-looking individual. He seems more amenable to solutions that are nontraditional in nature. I hope that his initiative is not completely subsumed by the Romanow one. I, of course, continue to have hopes for Mr. Romanow, and hope that he can manage a solid outcome in the time available.

I would go back to what I have said before: we're still in the relatively early stages of this debate. It's important to continue the dialogue. One way to do that is to continue to have these publicly sponsored reports. So I don't see these reports as negative. At some point we're going to have to move from the traditional "better system management" approaches to nontraditional "out-of-the-box" ones.

On a worldwide basis, the ideas we're discussing today aren't really outside the box. Of course, we cannot take another system and simply transplant it into Canada and say it is the right answer, but we can take elements of what's being done around the world and use them to improve our own system in a way that is consistent with Canadian values. Maybe these public discussions started by Romanow and others will help us at least look at that option.

DG: Fyke promotes primary health care reform and talks about it extensively in his report. Primary health care reform has become a staple in the speeches of ministers of health and premiers. The way motivational speakers talk about empowerment, politicians in Canada talk about primary care reform. What do you make of this idea?

WO: That depends on how you define it. For me, there are two elements of primary care reform that carry great promise: (1) information technology and (2) the use of teams.

As an industry, health care — and not just at the physician level — is grossly underinvested in terms of the use of information technology. One of the initiatives being discussed in Ontario is to link doctors through the creation of electronic medical records, thereby creating opportunity for access to laboratory results and other diagnostic testing results in a way that's compatible with what we should be doing in the twenty-first century. So information technology as an element to primary care reform is a great part of the process.

The other element involves teams. There are things that can be done as well or better by other health care providers that are currently being done by doctors. If we work in teams and we can allocate those tasks to the appropriate team members, we can make much more effective use of physicians' time.

But to look to primary care reform as the panacea for all of our problems is just not reasonable. In the greater scheme of things it's very unlikely to save money, but it hopefully will produce better-quality care and help us address the physician human resource issue by allowing physicians to leverage their time better.

DG: The two elements that you've mentioned are pretty noncontroversial. But there's a third element to primary health care reform: changing from a fee-for-service compensation for physicians to a capitation scheme. Proponents argue that this is the way to encourage physicians to spend more time with patients, while reducing costs and producing a more efficient system. What do you make of that argument?

WO: I don't believe that the fee-for-service system drives up health care costs. Physicians in Canada are so busy that the last thing they need to do is to look at how they can see more patients more often, and how they can increase the cost for an individual patient's care.

Fee-for-service has been around for a long time — 3,000 years or more in health care — and we ought to be pretty darn sure of what we're going to replace it with before we throw it out. Physicians should have choice in this issue, just as patients should have choice. Some physicians prefer to be remunerated in a salaried, capitated, or global model. I think they should have the freedom of choice.

Capitation will not replace fee-for-service. A blended system — what we're considering in Ontario — offers capitation for a basket of services, but fee-for-service for other services like hospital-based, emergency, and obstetrical services. But again, to suggest that physician compensation, narrowly defined as fee-for-service versus capitation, will somehow be the saviour of the business is, in my view, overly simplistic.

DG: You mentioned looking abroad. You've been clear that you don't look at the American system as particularly inviting for innovative ideas. Looking overseas, what do you see and what do you like?

WO: You mentioned some of the ideas earlier, like public-private partnerships.

I'm not convinced that the publicly funded system ought to cover all expenses [first-dollar coverage] or be the only insurer. Australia, for instance, encourages and subsidizes private insurance. Public and private services cooperate, often co-locating and sharing scarce resources such as MRIs. There is a symbiosis between the two and patients can choose. They have options. There are small, upfront user fees as well, in some circumstances.

In Holland, for instance, if you need a total joint arthroplasty, you get a promise that it will happen within a prescribed time period. If the public system can't provide it, you take your promissory certificate to the parallel private system and it will provide the procedure for you at no cost. Intriguing idea. Why shouldn't we at least look at that and see if there's some way we can put some pressure on the public system to perform better? One way to do it might be through Holland's kind of competitive environment.

There are ways of organizing and reorganizing, where we can find synergies between the public and the private systems to benefit everyone: patients, providers, and governments.

DG: There still isn't a politician today who talks about a parallel private system, or a more substantive role for the private sector, or anything that moves away from first-dollar coverage — which could be in the form of user fees or some form of medical savings accounts. Have we made progress, and where are we going?

WO: We've made huge progress. We came close in the last federal election campaign to having some level of discussion about this issue but it was impossible to sustain it beyond the leaders' debate. We need to continue that discussion now.

It should be impossible for a politician to avoid joining the debate. They can put it off for a while by creating commissions — like the one headed by Romanow — but as information continues to become available, as non-politicians and physician leaders and others continue to push the debate, and as authors like you continue to write award-winning books, I don't think they'll be able avoid it forever as pressures continue to build on providers and patients. Health care has shown great staying power as the number one front-of-mind issue for Canadians. Politicians will, of necessity, come on board.

I hope that that happens before there's more serious deterioration in the system, before it gets to the point where we can't rebuild it. I remain an optimist. I think we've made huge progress in the last two and a half years, which is a relatively brief time for a debate on a public policy of this significance. I'm hopeful.

LOW-TECH, LOW-BROW

Neil Seeman

In government reports, much ink is dedicated to the question of quality: are Canadians getting quality care? Often, the authors of these documents look to figures like physicians per capita and nurses per hospital bed to derive reassuring answers. Measuring the care available to patients involves more, however, than just comparing crude statistics. One basic criterion should be the ability of a health care system to offer patients proven, modern diagnostic tests and treatments. In his extensively researched essay, journalist and lawyer Neil Seeman looks at the technology available to Canadians.

Like others, he documents the dearth of diagnostic machinery. Seeman notes that Canada ranks 11th of 13 Organisation of Economic Co-Operation and Development (OECD) nations in terms of the availability of MRIs and 12th of 15 for CT scans. Seeman also observes the result of this deficiency, citing, for example, a study suggesting that Canadians wait about 150 days for an MRI scan, while Americans wait 3 days.

Such numbers, of course, fail to describe the quality of the equipment. Seeman finds a thirty-seven-year-old X-ray machine in a Montreal hospital and an ultrasound so obsolete that a Victoria hospital couldn't donate it to a local vet (the vet had better diagnostic equipment).

But Seeman goes much further. Exploring the latest advances in incontinence treatment, the diagnosis of irregular heartbeats, and the provision of cancer therapies, Seeman finds that Canadians get dated care. Moreover, in the case of the first example, patients have no access to a basic bladder-flow measurement device used everywhere else in the world. Nor do they have access to a leading therapeutic device — developed in Canada and subsidized by Canadian taxpayers — that indicates the early onset of heart attacks. The suffering endured by patients is, as Seeman bluntly describes, "gut wrenching." As well, there are implications for outcomes, particularly with regard to our aged diagnostic machinery: "Without quality diagnostic equipment available, one's prognosis for severely disabling illnesses — notably cancer — suffers." Ironically, long-term costs are often higher because of substandard treatments.

Not content to simply criticize, Seeman explores the reason for this technology gap. Drawing on the work of essayist W. Allen Wallis and economist Milton Friedman, Seeman argues that a government-run system has a disincentive to introduce new technologies. This fact draws Seeman to a profound conclusion: there must be an expanded role for private medicine in Canada. To bolster this claim, Seeman doesn't look south but, among other places, to Russia.

Seeman concludes: "Let's not fritter away life-saving technologies just because they don't fit into the Procrustean bed of medicare's budget. Let us embrace them; let us embrace the doctors who want to stay in Canada to use the new devices; let us embrace the entrepreneurs who want to help invent them. And let us embrace the millions of Canadians whose lives will be immeasurably enriched if we do."

Five dollars is all it takes to diagnose a bladder problem. And that's using the best technology in the world. The "Uroflow" Meter (or Urodyn 1000), developed by Medtronic Ltd.,[1] is widely used to benefit millions of seniors in rich and poor countries everywhere. Everywhere, that is, except Canada. The Uroflow is a special device that measures how much, and at what strength, a person urinates. Upon application, the physician can immediately diagnose a problem.

So why did this inexpensive, but inordinately useful invention — if you know anyone who suffers from urinary incontinence you know just how debilitating (and humiliating) the condition can be[2] — sell just a handful of units in Canada last year? Because Canadian physicians using this noninvasive device get reimbursed by provincial insurance plans at less than $4 per usage. That rate doesn't cover the cost of the disposal components, let alone the cost of the device itself (roughly $5,000) amortized over a period of several years. Hospital administrators aren't too thrilled about swallowing the shortfall. The result? Since urologists won't perform the simple diagnostic test in their offices, we end up clogging hospitals with patients waiting for a more invasive and more expensive test to be performed at a central facility. You don't need to be an economics major to know there's a problem here.

The Uroflow Meter is but one example of a worrying trend. Dozens of diagnostic and therapeutic products developed decades ago, in widespread use in other countries, are relatively unavailable to Canadians. Another example is the SynchroMed implantable drug infusion pump, a therapeutic device that, when combined with an antispasmodic drug, can be used in patients with severe spasticity resulting from injury (spinal cord trauma, brain injury) or disease (multiple sclerosis, cerebral palsy) to regain their mobility and independence, and to control their pain.[3] Patients using SynchroMed, from war-ravaged Yugoslavia to fiscally-racked Russia, save their respective health care systems upwards of $100,000 per year in treatment costs. Meanwhile, Canadian hospitals refuse to provide patients with the $8,000 device.[4]

Not one to pull his punches, Vern Dale-Johnson, the director of Medtronic of Canada Ltd., finds this both economically puzzling and morally absurd:

> Our health ministries, in Ontario and elsewhere across Canada, are reluctant to spend the $8,000 for a pump, support the infrastructure needed (nurse clinicians for refills and follow-up and appropriate OR time), and supply the $2,000 per year in liquid baclofen required through the hospital pharmacy. Instead we ask patients and their families to suffer and struggle through a life of pain and torment caused by severe muscle spasticity and by the relinquishing [of] control and support to chronic care institutions, costing, you will find, well over $100,000 per patient per year . . .[5]

This predicament produces dozens, perhaps hundreds, of casualties every year. The most infamous case: Tracy Latimer. "The media misses the issue," says Dale-Johnson. He goes on:

> The question should be, "Why did the Saskatchewan health care mosaic fail Tracy Latimer and her family? Why was the only option given to the family one more painful, destructive surgical procedure when an alternate procedure was available that would have relieved both the pain and the severe spasticity that trapped Tracy in her body?" . . . If the Saskatchewan health minister could be held responsible for the actions of the Ministry, he would have been on trial along with Robert Latimer as an accessory to murder.[6]

It's a debate that tugs at the emotions.

"Reveal" is a finger-sized, $2,000 device that is considered the "gold standard" for diagnosing patients with palpitations that may suggest the onset of cardiac arrhythmia, the condition that afflicts U.S. Vice-President

Dick Cheney and former NBA superstar and U.S. Presidential Candidate Bill Bradley. Even though it's made in Canada, with Canadian parts, Reveal is easier to find in places like Kosovo and Kalamazoo than in Vancouver or Toronto. Also troubling is the fact that Reveal was developed with the assistance of Canadian taxpayers, who subsidized its production and distribution costs courtesy of one of the Liberal government's myriad programs to boost homegrown high-tech.[7]

Canada has a lower purchasing rate of Reveal than any other industrial country. Instead of spending $2,000 on Reveal, which can stop fainting spells and arrhythmia-induced seizures cold, Canadian hospitals will spend tens of thousands of dollars every year on screening tests followed by electrophysiology. A typical large hospital in Toronto might see ten patients suffering from arrhythmia-induced seizures in a given year. Instead of spending the $40,000 to treat those ten patients with a Reveal — $20,000 plus the cost of surgery — hospitals will typically spend $4 million on tests and various treatments. None of that, of course, considers the cost to an employer, and to society, of harbouring people who could faint or fall onto the floor or onto their steering wheels without warning.

Wait a second, you're probably thinking, what about all those "centres of excellence" everyone's always talking about? Chances are you've heard it said that "Canada has the best health care system in the world." Surely a "centre of excellence" in a country that boasts the "best health care system in the world" can scrounge up enough cash to stop a bout of fainting spells or treat a bursting bladder or help a spasmodic child? Sadly, no.

Consider what is Canada's best known "centre of excellence": the Hospital for Sick Children in downtown Toronto. Even though it is widely recognized as Canada's leading treatment centre for young children — which it indubitably is — it falls down in crucial areas. Like spasticity (involuntary jerking motions, secondary to a neurological condition). Sick Kids' Hospital is without a specialized spasticity program; few pediatric hospitals, *public or private*, in major American cities *anywhere* are without such a program. What is more, provincial insurance plans won't pay for implantable pumps to control spasticity in children. *Public* insurance in almost every industrialized country everywhere else in the world covers such devices, even in a country like the U.S., which has a healthy marketplace in private medicine. All of which means that children in Canada who suffer from spasticity — generally as a result of brain injury or cerebral palsy — must pay for these items themselves, and then must strain to lobby beneficent doctors and administrators to have the surgery done. This is a Sisyphean task, especially considering that parents of children with such maladies have no central voice; to the extent that they belong to groups that represent their interests,[8] these groups exist mainly to lobby for research into a cure, not to advocate for better therapeutic treatment.

Left to their own devices, patients limp laboriously through medicare's Byzantine rules. "First you have to convince the Canadian specialists that they aren't always offering the best treatments here, and that can be difficult," says Gerald Ray, a seventy-four-year-old Toronto man who went to England several years ago for an effective new treatment for cancer of the soft palate. Photodynamic therapy is standard treatment in England, but is not available in Canada.[9] A similar experience befell the parents of Lance Relland, an Alberta teenager with an aggressive cancer known as lymphoblastic leukemia. Lance was ultimately fortunate enough to undergo bone marrow treatment at the University of Minnesota. "In some cases, they are handing a death sentence to the patients," says Charles Relland, commenting on the way Canadian hospital administrators handle cases like his son's. Lance has now recovered and resumed life as a university student.

Cases like Lance Relland's are gut wrenching, so much so that they may conceivably bias the terms of debate over medicare reform. "We must see the forest, not the trees," insist medicare's defenders. After all, high-tech medicine may not be a panacea. Consider the words of leading medicare apologist Dr. Michael Rachlis, a Toronto activist and the author of two books on Canadian health care: "If you're simply getting a better image of something but it doesn't change any of the subsequent management, then you haven't improved anybody's health."[10]

To be sure, many of the hospitals that make *U.S. News & World Report*'s annual list of "best hospitals" often do so using a "low-tech" approach to medicine. An influential 1999 Yale University study in the *New England Journal of Medicine* found that surprisingly low-tech medical treatment — such as the use of aspirins and beta blockers — was the trademark of a great many top-rated cardiac care facilities.[11] This is a trenchant observation, but heart disease and spasticity are as similar as chalk and cheese. Heart disease affects a broad and vocal constituency; spasticity affects a tiny and quiescent one.[12]

Canadian politicians are mindful of these disparities when running for office and debating the politics of medicare. In his classic analysis of political entrepreneurship, *An Overgoverned Society*, W. Allen Wallis notes that one of the ways that politicians compete for votes is by offering to have the government provide new services.[13] Yet, for an offer of a "new" service to have substantial electoral impact, the service ordinarily must be one that a large number of voters is familiar with, and in fact already use. The most effective innovations for a political entrepreneur to offer, therefore, are those in which it is possible to transfer the costs of services already in existence from individuals to the government without appreciably altering the amount of the services that reach the people. For this reason, medicare carries an inherent bias against the provision of innovative services and procedures. Provincial reimbursement plans are loath to add new treatments of narrow electoral benefit to the list of covered items; the same logic applies to diagnostics, which get updated by provincial listing authorities once every ten years.

Expanding on Wallis's theory of political entrepreneurship, the economist and Nobel laureate Milton Friedman recently observed that "once the bulk of costs have been taken over by government . . . the political entrepreneur has no additional groups to attract, and attention turns to holding down costs."[14] This, in a nutshell, is the operating ethos of hospital administrators across Canada.[15]

Wallis's theory of political entrepreneurship explains why broad-impact illnesses like heart disease have enjoyed exponentially more research funding than have illnesses like childhood spasticity. And so we are years, if not decades, away from treating spasticity with the "low-tech" analog of beta blockers. Until then, should we refrain from treating childhood spasticity with available but expensive pain-relieving implantation devices, anguished parents will continue to strap hockey helmets on their head-banging children. Incredibly, such is Canada's preferred treatment protocol for childhood spasticity.

◆

In actuality, Canada does not enjoy anything like the best health care system in the world. And it is a truism that bears repeating that Canada's is the "best health care system in the world" only until such time as you or one of your loved ones falls ill. The only way Canada's health care system can lift itself out of perdition is to embrace new technologies, which necessarily means embracing private care. In an essay for the *National Post*, Queen's University economist Thomas Courchene put it thus:

... the real challenge is not how to keep the private sector out of health; rather, it is how to bring it in! The essential point is that we cannot allow the last paradigm's conception of medicare to prevent the health sector from emerging as a pivotal player in our society. . . . If we fail in making the health sector a viable economic platform for human capital and knowledge-based enterprise, then the sector will likewise fail in providing state-of-the-art health care.[16]

Courchene's is the lesson now being learned in Russia, where private hospitals like MedSanChast in Moscow are the only facilities in the nation with sufficient funds available to pay for European machines to analyze blood for venereal disease and to diagnose the life-threatening septic illnesses that are ravaging the Russian countryside. Were it not for these new private hospitals and the burgeoning middle class that is paying their freight, poorer Russians attending nearby public facilities would not benefit from the growing spillover in treatment methodologies, and many of the public health problems now searing the country might have no end in sight.

Sadly, neo-Russian capitalism has yet to catch on in socialist Canada. Consider what Health Minister Allan Rock told the journal *Health Affairs* in June 2000: "I'm determined to maintain the current public system, not out of stale dogma or rigid catechism, but because I believe profoundly that it is the best from the social perspective and also makes the most economic sense."[17]

This is a truly breathtaking statement coming from the minister of health, who presumably must abide by basic facts to form his opinions. We know from data collated by the Fraser Institute that the median time needed to wait for radiation oncology in Canada is now nine weeks.[18] By any rational economic measure, waiting lists are an ineffective way for a health care system to manage costs. The longer an employee is away from work, the less likely it is that she will return. The 2000 figures from Ontario's Workplace Safety and Insurance Board show that if a thirty-five-year-old carpenter earning $3,000 a month has been disabled for a year, more than $160,000 in reserves must be set aside for the worker's pension if he never returns to work. Finally, a six-week delay in radiation oncology may mean the difference between a benign tumour metastasizing from the ear into the brain — the difference, that is, between life and death.

And it's not just money at stake. In 1997, 121 Ontario residents were removed from the list for coronary-artery bypass grafts because their condition deteriorated to the point that they became medically unfit for surgery.

This deterioration happened while they were waiting for treatment. And according to a report released in fall 2000 by the Canadian Association of Radiologists, your radiological diagnosis may be proven wrong by the time you end up in the specialist's office! According to the study, up to half of all radiological machines in Canada, from ultrasounds to CT scanners, are either dilapidated or obsolete.

Frustrated by the Third World conditions in their midst, hundreds of Canadian radiologists abandon the country every year to practise in the United States or Europe.[19] The poor quality of Canada's medical equipment was most poignantly illustrated recently when a Cambodian refugee camp rejected a free ultrasound machine from a top hospital in Victoria because it was antediluvian. Just to raise the standard of treatment and diagnostics to minimally acceptable standards will require an infusion of at least $1 billion, according to the radiologists' association.

A flood of statistics now shows that Canada lags behind most members of the Organisation for Economic Co-Operation and Development (OECD) with regard to medical equipment.[20] Recent reports have indicated that magnetic resonance imaging (MRI) machines and computed tomography (CT) scanners across the country are falling apart. Canada ranks 12th among 15 OECD nations in terms of the availability of CT scanners — behind poorer countries such as Korea, Portugal, and Spain. In terms of MRIs, Canada ranks 11th out of 13 — just a hair ahead of Poland. Last year, one Montreal hospital was reportedly using a thirty-seven-year-old X-ray machine that is only supposed to last twelve years. At another hospital, a CT scanner bore an ominous sign: "Do Not Shut Down." Technologists had apparently found that if it was turned off, they could not start it back up again.

Shortages have already led to an "unconscionable" delay in the diagnosis and treatment of diseases such as cancer, heart disease, and debilitating bone and joint ailments, according to an assessment given in 2000 by the Canadian Medical Association (CMA). Thousands of Canadians suffer physical pain and emotional anxiety while they wait for their diagnosis. Some die because it's too late to treat their disease by the time it is finally diagnosed, and even rudimentary medical equipment is woefully in short supply. "We're not talking about Ferraris and Lamborghinis here," says Dr. Hugh Scully, the CMA head. "We're talking about the Chevrolets and the Fords that are necessary to make it [diagnosis] accessible and reasonable for everybody."[21]

Dr. John Radomsky, president of the Canadian Association of Radiologists, told *Southam News* that it is common for patients with excruciating lower back pain to be forced to wait for as long as eight months for an MRI to determine whether surgery is necessary. "That's unconscionable. In most countries, you can get in within a week or two. Why should we accept months of pain, when in many cases, we don't need to?" he asked.[22]

A recent study by the Fraser Institute found that although Canada is 5th highest among the 29 OECD countries in spending on health as a percentage of GDP, it is generally among the bottom third in terms of the availability of medical technology. It found Canada was 21st of 28 OECD nations in availability of CT scanners, 19th of 22 in availability of lithotriptors (used to treat kidney stones and gallstones), and 19th of 27 in availability of MRIs. Canada ranked 6th of 17 in availability of radiation equipment.[23]

"People who might otherwise either have their life extended or have their life saved are not getting that kind of leading-edge treatment because we have not made the commitment to acquire the latest technologies," says Michael Walker, executive director of the Fraser Institute. A comparison of technology also found that CT scanners, nuclear medicine facilities, MRIs, lithotriptors, position emission tomography (PET) machines, specialized intensive care facilities, and cardiac catheter labs are all much less likely to be found at a community hospital in British Columbia than at a similar hospital in Washington or Oregon. As well, angioplasty and transplant facilities are restricted mainly to university teaching hospitals in British Columbia, while they are far more widely dispersed in the two American states.

To insouciantly ignore these realities, as does Ottawa's current Liberal government, requires a breathtaking arrogance or callousness, or both.

Pace Mr. Rock, it is both economically and morally unsound to defend the status quo. It is wrong to prohibit sick people from seeking immediate, potentially life-saving diagnosis and treatment. And it is wrong for parents to plead with hospital administrators to bend medicare's rules to find treatment for their sick children. But that is the way things will remain unless medicare brooks a major, radical overhaul. Better yet — an implosion.

Under the current regime, hospital administrators have only two motivations: (1) to balance their global budgets, set in January of each year and (2) to have their facility become known as a "centre of excellence." In order to meet either goal, it is imperative that hospitals contain costs and refrain from experimental, expensive procedures. Chances are you've heard about how all those bean-counting M.B.A.s at health maintenance organizations

(HMOs) throughout the United States limit or "cap" what types of proce-dures doctors are allowed to perform. The same thing happens in Canada, but it is so commonplace that we accept it unquestioningly. Just ask Ron Kramer, a Canadian businessman who sought treatment for esophageal cancer in the United States because the American procedure posted much better survival rates than the method offered north of the border. The Ontario Health Insurance Plan (OHIP), citing the American method as experimental, refuses to fund the $342,000 procedure.

"This [system] compels people to either choose economy and die here or go to the States and live," says Richard Shekter, Mr. Kramer's lawyer, who has handled a number of such medical denial cases. "Nobody is going to acknowledge publicly that they are providing second-class medicine," he told the *National Post*. "But this isn't a once-in-a-lifetime rare procedure, this is generalized treatment of esophageal cancer. It is a generic issue and it means they are not doing their job." For doctors, he says, "it means that you'd have to acknowledge to every patient who walked in with esophageal cancer we practise substandard, sub-quality medicine. You can get better medicine in the States. Get out of here. They won't do it."[24]

For Canadian physicians to refuse to acknowledge the palpable limita-tions of medicare is a breach of their Hippocratic oath. And yet, their behaviour is understandable. Recommending that their patients go south to the United States, or that they visit a private clinic in Canada in order to obtain expedited treatment, is anathema to many doctors. This attitude stems in part from a kind of sunny devotion to medicare that is inculcated first in medical school and later, by one's peers, in practice. It also stems from the strictures and loopholes presented by the Canada Health Act. The Act, though it ostensibly brooks private enterprise and private health insurance — an oft-misunderstood and misreported fact — explicitly forbids anyone from buying from the private sector any medical service that is already covered under the public health system.

As a matter of law, the prohibition is vague. While it clearly allows public hospitals to contract with private firms under a global budget, as was envi-sioned in the early drafts of Alberta's "Bill 11,"[25] it is not at all clear that it allows private individuals to pay more than is stipulated under provincial reimbursement plans for any given treatment.[26] This is a key point because, again as a matter of law, the issue of whether a surgery performed without waiting is deemed the same "treatment" as surgery for which one is required to wait months, has never been litigated.[27] It is my opinion that these things are not coequal, meaning that Canadians should be allowed, under the current law, to pay cash for quicker access to key surgeries performed in the private sector. The trouble is, until such time as this issue is resolved in court or by Parliament, no private clinic wants to be a legal test case. And so, for all intents and purposes, the prohibition on private medicine is real.[28]

The consequences of this state of affairs are profound. With an aging population, medicare will be judged increasingly by its ability to expeditiously improve the quality of life of the old[29] and the infirm.[30] And all the early signs show that Canada is failing to deliver the type of care that seniors need and desire. A recent study by the Heart & Stroke Foundation of Canada found that although the number of heart attack deaths is steadily declining in Canada, the quality of life for survivors is worsening. This means that there is more to dealing with heart disease than simply providing sufferers with clot-busting drugs. Combine this fact with a study released in 2000 showing that the ischemia (poor cardiac blood flow) of only 54 percent of Canadian heart attack patients was improved by surgery or drug treatment (compared with 69 percent of U.S. patients), and you have one angry group of heart disease sufferers. Having grown up in a cohort that is used to getting what it wants, aging baby boomers, as Regina E. Herzlinger of Harvard Business School first observed,[31] will simply not abide by second-tier pain modalities.[32] Result: If they can't find the service they demand in Canada, they will simply fly south of the border to get it.[33]

Judging by the first ministers' health accord last fall, there is a growing recognition among Canadian politicians that medicare needs to confront the technology gap. In a presentation notable for its rare admission of some of the troubles afflicting medicare, Mr. Rock, before a gathering in Saskatoon in August 2000, outlined a general, seven-point proposal to address such issues as outdated medical equipment, information technology, and the brain drain of young doctors to the United States. His solution? A $500 million commitment to "Health Information Technology."

It is, of course, a paltry sum. More disturbing than the amount, however, is the ideology that undergirds it. Information technology cannot be willed into existence by government edict; only the private sector can fill the gap. Equally muddle-headed is the Liberal government's insistence on promoting "health information" rather than ushering in top-tier diagnostic equipment through the private marketplace.[34] "Information technology" is Liberal code for putting health data onto smart cards, which necessarily will require a new, large, and intrusive government bureaucracy to administer it.

✦

Medicare would be wise to focus less on centralized information gathering and more on spiriting new advances in medical technology. By any reasonable assessment, the Canadian system has abjured modern technology. Canadians wait an average of 150 days for an MRI scan; Americans, just 3. Canada has fewer MRI scanners — fifty-three — relative to its population than South Korea.[35] The current system "costs" some $100 billion a year, but that figure leaves out the tens of millions of dollars in disability costs and lost wages due to missed work. The consequences move far beyond economics, however. To save costs, Canadian surgeons often resort to traditional angiography as opposed to magnetic resonance angiography. Yet traditional angiography is a more hazardous procedure — the doctor must pass a fine tube into a femoral vessel in the fold of the groin while the patient is exposed to potentially toxic X-ray radiation — than safer MR imaging. Other invasive and often outdated medical procedures (such as lumbar puncture and orthoscopic knee surgery) are the price this country pays for its dearth of MRIs and other advanced technology. It also means that state-of-the-art MRI screening procedures — used in the early detection of breast cancer, for example[36] — are not available.[37]

Without quality diagnostic equipment available, one's prognosis for severely disabling illnesses — notably cancer — suffers. "We are already seeing serious disparities in incidence and mortality rates between Canada and the U.S. (according to the National Association of Central Cancer Registries) in the four major cancer sites," notes Beth Kapusta, the executive director of the Cancer Advocacy Coalition of Canada.[38] "That is to say, we are falling further and further behind, as doctors have more and more reasons [to leave] as they can't practise high-standard medicine [in Canada]."[39]

This is not a problem we can micromanage out of existence. Notwithstanding my opinion that a strong legal case can be made to show that medicare has broken its promise (a.k.a. contract) to Canadians, it would be wrong to try to fix the current morass via the courts. At the time of writing, the Canadian Association of Radiologists had just solicited a legal opinion that advised doctors to inform patients in advance of unreliable and outdated equipment, lest they be sued. "It is imperative that the patient be advised and understand the risks and uncertainties associated with the reliability of such an examination," wrote lawyer Chantal Corriveau of Montreal's Kugler Kandestin law firm.[40]

"The importance of 'shopping around' for treatment and diagnostic options is increasing," observes Kapusta. "The Canadian government refuses either to establish meaningful benchmarks for the cancer-care system, or to acknowledge that faulty equipment and delays are at fault in unnecessary deaths. One suspects that many of these cases will play out in the courts, not in the hospitals, as increasingly savvy patients understand the implications of delay and second-rate procedures, based on opinions received in the U.S. and standards of care available elsewhere in the world."[41]

As attractive as a favourable ruling from the courts might be, however, it would only signal a short-term solution. It would simply force the government to pay for a raft of new medical procedures without offering a sensible way for it to find the money to afford them. Exponentially higher federal taxes would almost certainly ensue. Nor is there any guarantee that the current Supreme Court of Canada, even in the teeth of overwhelming evidence of medicare's demise, would issue a judgment that essentially tells the government, "Your health system is broken." The bench is more liberal in ideology than it has been in quite some time, even under the generally level-headed stewardship of Madame Justice Beverly McLachlin. It is also politically dangerous for the medical establishment to position itself as the adversary of government. Finally, bringing suit would tempt doctors to practise "defensive medicine," whereby they eschew treating patients altogether rather than use machines that might be second-rate. Ethically, this is not the right gambit for medical professionals, who are honour-bound to advocate for the best possible care, not the best possible insulation from trial lawyers.

But "radiologists are not hiding behind a legal opinion, they are taking their responsibility very seriously and they're very concerned about patients," Dr. Normand Laberge, CEO of the Canadian Association of Radiologists, told the *Globe and Mail* earlier this year.[42] In the past several months, some of Dr. Laberge's machines have been deemed so useless that (a) Haiti, (b) an equine veterinarian, and (c) the aforementioned Cambodian refugee camp, have all turned them down although they were offered free of charge. Another radiologist, Toronto doctor Mark Prieditis, said his colleagues are wont to cope with an antiquated machine by "kicking it on the side or using duct tape, or turning it off and on ten times until it finally turns on." In Prince Albert, SK, Dr. Holy Wells reports that both of her hospital's fluoroscopy machines "die on a regular basis" so she is forced to ration barium enemas, a test to help detect colon cancer. At the Queen Elizabeth II

Health Sciences Centre, the largest training and referral centre in Atlantic Canada, almost 45 percent of imaging equipment needs replacing, according to Dr. Paul LeBrun, chief of imaging.[43] On Prince Edward Island, cancer treatment technology consists of a twenty-five-year-old cobalt therapy unit, and there is no diagnostic MRI. All the way over on Canada's other coast, Dr. Phil Malpass, a general practitioner in British Columbia's Kootenays, describes his practice environment thus:

> Since the early 1990s we've been facing many obstacles. Our 1954 hospital is dilapidated and termed "functionally obsolete," as is our long-term care hospital, Mount St. Francis. Equipment, including a secondhand fluoroscopic unit for pacemaker insertion and a 1947 autoclave for sterilizing debris, is frequently broken. We do not even have access to standard technology, like a CT scanner, which makes a huge difference in diagnosing certain conditions. Faced with surgical and internal medicine calls, at times covering the whole West Kootenay region, we are poorly equipped to meet the needs and expectations of our patients, but we do our best. Indeed this may be our downfall.[44]

Rationing. Fixing primitive technology. Defensive medicine. Physicians were trained for none of these things. Nor are these the types of things that we particularly want to send them to medical school to learn — at taxpayers' expense. Meanwhile, the overriding message to the patient on the state of Canadian technology has become "Consumer Beware," says Beth Kapusta. According to Kapusta, it is now "increasingly clear that those providing cancer services, from government down to the cancer agencies, are increasingly unable to act in the interests of the public good."[45] Both Kapusta and Doug Hitchlock, the president of the Free Trade Medical Network Inc. in Toronto, point to a short-term strategy to help staunch the haemorrhage: timely public reimbursement for diagnostic services that are available, without delay, outside the country.

Hitchlock (with whom I work at Free Trade Medical) is a stockbroker of forty years' experience who left Bay Street to start a health information and diagnostic referral company in Toronto after his nine-year-old daughter died on a waiting list for angioplasty. He thinks the official Liberal policy of discouraging Canadians from purchasing premium quality services south of the border is bizarre, to say the least. "If you needed a ride, and your country had a shortage of buses, but plenty of bus stations, would you sit around for ten years until the buses were built? Would you cross your fingers and hope that the government might some day cough up enough money to build the buses? Or would you go south of the border, where they build the best buses in the world, and jump on a bus to get from A to B?" asks Hitchlock, audibly exasperated.[46]

To borrow Dr. Malpass's phrase, medicare is "functionally obsolete" when it comes to equipping Canadian hospitals with adequate tools to do the job, much less state-of-the-art technology. That is a painful reality. It is simply intellectually dishonest to deny it. Nor does accepting this fact — and embracing private sector alternatives — mean that Canada will lose its identity as a distinct nation known far and wide to care for the indigent and the downtrodden. Quite the opposite. Modern medicine is expensive. Each new discovery, medication, diagnostic machine, or operating device costs a great deal. For example, the cost of the additional equipment to perform laparoscopic gallbladder removals — the cameras, televisions, and laparoscopes — typically exceeds $100,000. The new neurosurgical equipment that will use computers to assist in brain surgery will cost upwards of $1 million. An MRI generally costs $1 million.[47] That is a fraction of the amount of money that Ottawa and the provinces have spent on CCOHTA (rhymes with quota), the Soviet-sounding "Canadian Coordinating Office for Health Technology Assessment."

Set up in 1989, CCOHTA's mandate is to assess the pros and cons of allowing medicare to pay for new medical technologies. Dr. Renaldo Battista — head of CCOHTA's Quebec counterpart, l'Agence d'Evaluation de Technologie et des Modes d'Intervention en Santé — sums up the situation using the story of Icarus, who, to escape the Minotaur's labyrinth with his father Daedalus, flew too close to the sun. The glue on his artificial wings melted and Icarus fell into the sea. "In order to contain the dreaded beast of illness and death, we have come to build a very intricate labyrinth, the health care system," Dr. Battista said. "At this point in time, we all feel, to some extent, trapped in this labyrinth. We don't know exactly what is the way out, what are the solutions. We see the problems but we can't seem to figure out what are the ultimate solutions."[48]

Organizations like CCOHTA *are* the problem. Let's not fritter away life-saving technologies just because they don't fit into the Procrustean bed of medicare's budget. Let us embrace them; let us embrace the doctors who want to stay in Canada to use the new devices; let us embrace the entrepreneurs who want to help invent them. And let us embrace the millions of Canadians whose lives will be immeasurably enriched if we do.

96 * BETTER MEDICINE

1. The company's headquarters is in Minneapolis, MN.
2. Roughly 500,000 Canadians suffer from bladder dysfunction. Many of these patients are too embarrassed by potential leakage and the odour of urine to set foot outside their doors. Another implantable device, the Interstim Sacral Nerve Stimulation System, has been found to lower rates of suicide in people suffering from urinary incontinence. Interstim has been on the market in Canada since 1994, but few doctors or centres in Canada offer the procedure for two reasons: (1) there are not many physicians trained in its insertion method and (2) the cost, at $7,000 to $10,000, is prohibitive.
3. Surgeons insert the pump under the abdominal skin. It's then connected to an elastic catheter that delivers medication directly to the intrathecal space (the area surrounding the spinal cord). The pump needs to be refilled by a nurse every four to six weeks. The Health Protection Branch has approved the pump, but due to decreasing hospital budgets, it is rarely available.
4. When you account for the implantable life of the pump, it costs less than $1,500 per year.
5. Vern Dale-Johnson, interview, Mississauga, ON, 29 Jan. 2001.
6. Ibid.
7. Specifically, Industrial Research Assistance Program.
8. Cerebral Palsy Association of Canada, Heart & Stroke Foundation of Canada, Parkinson's Foundation of Canada, and so on.
9. T. Arnold, "It's More Than Just Funding," *National Post*, 7 Feb. 2001, A13.
10. M. Kennedy, "MDs Want $1.74B High-Tech Injection: Canada's Shortage of Equipment Leads to 'Unconscionable' Delays in Diagnosis — CT-scans More Accessible in Portugal, Korea and Spain," *Ottawa Citizen*, 21 May 2000, A1.
11. J. Chen et al., "Do 'America's Best Hospitals' Perform Better for Acute Myocardial Infarction?" *New England Journal of Medicine*, 340.4 (28 Jan. 1999): 286–94.
12. Heart disease killed an estimated 79,100 Canadians last year [2000]; spasticity, though severely debilitating, affected just hundreds Canadian children last year.
13. W. Allen Wallis, *An Overgoverned Society* (New York: Free Press, 1976), 256.
14. M. Friedman, "How to Cure Health Care," *The Public Interest* 142 (Winter 2001): 32.
15. Indeed, Dr. Hugh Scully, the president of the Canadian Medical Association, has said that medicare likely cannot survive without limits on the services it offers.
16. T. Courchene, "Smart Money Well Spent," *National Post*, 11 Jan. 2001, A18.
17. J.K. Inglehart, "Restoring the Status of an Icon: A Talk with Canada's Minister of Health," *Health Affairs*, May/June 2000, 137.
18. M. Walker and G. Wilson, *Waiting Your Turn: Hospital Waiting Lists in Canada* (Vancouver: The Fraser Institute, 2000), 37. Although Fraser Institute data are routinely impugned for not being "peer-reviewed" by medicare apologists (notably Toronto activist Michael Rachlis and University of Toronto health administration professor Raisa Deber), they remain the only data anywhere in Canada that address the subject of waiting lists in a reliable and consistent manner. As for their veracity, it is hard to conceive why thousands of Canadian medical specialists, who annually provide the Fraser Institute with the requisite information in a transparent manner, would have any incentive to fudge these statistics. For a further analysis of the Fraser Institute study and comparisons with more selective data, see Chapter 1 in David

Gratzer, *Code Blue: Reviving Canada's Health Care System* (Toronto: ECW Press, 1999), 19–58.

19. Canada loses approximately four to five graduating medical school classes every year to the United States.

20. Arnold, "It's More Than Just Funding."

21. M. Kennedy, "Doctors Plead for Diagnostic Machines: MRI, CT Scanners Needed," *National Post/Southam News*, 22 May 2000, A9.

22. Ibid.

23. See M. Zelder, *Spend More, Wait Less? The Myth of Underfunded Medicare in Canada* (Vancouver: The Fraser Institute, 2000). Available on the Internet at www.fraserinstitute.ca/publications/forum/2000/08/.

24. Arnold, "It's More Than Just Funding."

25. Although press reports invariably note that Bill 11 would "expand the role of the private sector" in Alberta, this is a false assumption. Under its current iteration, Bill 11 would, in fact, roll back the aegis of the private sector by imposing $10,000 to $20,000 fines on legal private clinics throughout the province.

26. This lacuna in the law was implicitly conceded by Monique Bégin, the former Liberal health minister and architect of the 1984 Canada Health Act, when, in May 2000, she reentered the political fray to call upon Ottawa to draft a law that would explicitly forbid the increasing privatization of medicare.

27. Canada's first ministers have conceded as much. The language of the first ministers' $23.4 billion health accord in September 2000 promised to provide Canadians with only "reasonably timely" access to health care. But the Canada Health Act speaks of "access," not "reasonable" access. The weaselly word "reasonable" has become a favourite of late among staunch defenders of medicare like Toronto activist Michael Rachlis and Raisa Deber of the University of Toronto, who have suggested that medicare never promised Canadians "access," only "reasonable access." This is both historically false and disingenuous.

28. See C. Flood and T. Archibald, "The Illegality of Private Health Care in Canada," *Canadian Medical Association Journal* 164.6 (2001): 825–30. Analyzing multiple layers of provincial regulation, the authors conclude: "Private insurance for medically necessary hospital and physician services is illegal in only 6 of the 10 provinces. *Nonetheless, a significant private sector has not developed in any of the 4 provinces that do permit private insurance coverage.* The absence of a significant private sector is probably best explained by the prohibitions on the subsidy of private practice by public plans, measures that prevent physicians from topping up their public sector incomes with private fees." (Emphasis mine.)

29. According to a 2000 report by the Canadian Medical Association, in twenty-five years seniors will represent 21 percent of the Canadian population and will account for about 60 percent ($112 billion) of health care spending. Drug costs will soar from $4 billion to more than $15 billion in 2026, the CMA report predicted. For more on demographics and health costs, see David Baxter's essay in this volume.

30. The Canadian-born social commentator Malcolm Gladwell made this point in an influential debate last year with fellow expatriate Adam Gopnik, published in the *Washington Monthly* ("Canada v. U.S.: A Health Care Debate Between Adam Gopnik and Malcolm Gladwell," *The Washington Monthly* 22 [Mar. 2000]: 25–37). Gladwell paints the difference between post-operative care in the U.S. and Canada as follows: ". . . the issue is not mortality; it's morbidity. If you look at the levels of suffering, if

you look at the guy who is 68 years old and has got blocked arteries, in America that guy gets a bypass and his level of how active he is, whether he's going to work, whether he's playing golf twice a day, the American is way better off. Take a 72-year-old Canadian with severe angina. He does not get a bypass. The American, he gets a bypass in a week! . . . The Canadian system has no problem inconveniencing the family and fundamentally inconveniencing the employer."

31. R.E. Herzlinger, *Market-Driven Health Care: Who Wins, Who Loses in the Transformation of America's Largest Service Industry* (Cambridge: Addison-Wesley, 1997).

32. New surveys reveal how prescient this observation was. A 2000 poll by Angus Reid found that 58 percent of Canadians believe medicare should cover only "core services." That was a milestone in Canadian public opinion; a clear majority of Canadians now accept the logic of having two tiers, one private and one public. The proportion might be higher than 58 percent because Angus Reid's question may have repelled respondents who favoured pure, market-oriented remedies, such as RSP-like medical savings accounts. For more on medical savings accounts, see David Gratzer's essay in this volume.

33. Figures regarding how much money Canadians spend on health care south of the border are notoriously hard to come by. Less than 0.1 percent of Canadians reported being treated in the U.S. in the past year in the 1998–99 National Population Health Survey. However, the federal Liberals have released no definitive information since 1997, when, based on 1993 data, Health Canada reported that Canadians spend $1 billion on U.S. health care annually. The Fraser Institute puts the figure at twice that amount. The actual figure may be closer to $20 billion. New data collected by the Cancer Advocacy Coalition of Canada (www.canceradvocacy.com) reveal an exploding, multibillion dollar industry in cross-border medical shopping. Regarding the confusion surrounding these figures, author David Frum has observed, "The failure to collect information is one reason for medicare's famously low administrative costs. But it is also one of the reasons for medicare's famous insensitivity to patient well-being. . . . Medicare fails to gather information because — as a government monopoly — it does not need it." See D. Frum, "Ordinary Joes Know Medicare's Woes," *National Post*, 27 Nov. 1999, B10.

34. Perhaps the most jejune of all proposals cast about in the medicare debate is the need for health care "report cards." Although unobjectionable in theory, it is seldom mentioned that the government agencies charged with vetting such reports (namely, the Canadian Institute for Health Information) place value on competition among regions, but not among hospitals. From the patient's perspective, knowing how hospital A differs from hospital B in one's home town is vastly more important than knowing the aggregate differences in quality between Prince Edward Island and British Columbia. Without interhospital competition fostered by private care, however, hospitals have no incentive to publish such information.

35. According to data provided by the Montreal-based Canadian Association of Radiologists, there are only fifty-three MRIs in all of Canada, and the distribution varies among the provinces. Ontario has the most with twenty-three, Quebec has ten, B.C. has nine (including two that are privately owned), and Alberta has six. Saskatchewan, Manitoba, Nova Scotia, New Brunswick, and Newfoundland each have one. In October 1998, a joint committee of Alberta Health officials and regional health authorities announced that if the province doubled the number of MRI scans — from 30,000 to 60,000 — it would bring Alberta up to the level of a conservative U.S. HMO in 1992.

36. An even more state-of-the art diagnostic methodology for breast cancer — using computer graphics designed for NASA — is available in the U.S. but is decades from being introduced into Canada. Preliminary studies by scientists at the University of Pennsylvania, aimed to enhance mammograms using this digital 3-D mammography equipment, suggest the "space age" approach may decrease false-positive rates by 50 percent. See "Hi-Tech Imaging Could Cut Biopsy Rate," *Medical Post,* 20 Jan. 1998, A1.

37. MRI is also increasingly being used to investigate vascular disease. Unlike angiography for such investigations, MRI is noninvasive and is a much less complicated procedure to perform. In October 1999, doctors at the University of Mississippi Medical Center reported that MRI-guided cryosurgery was a promising way to destroy renal tumours.

38. Study released Nov. 16, 2000 (cf. www.naacr.org). The study poignantly concludes: "Canadians with some types of cancer may not do as well as their counterparts in some U.S. states — even when adjustments are made for varying incidence rates."

39. The high-tech staffing crisis will grow as increasing numbers leave for the U.S. or retire. According to Normand Laberge, CEO of the Canadian Association of Radiologists, the average age of Canadian radiologists is now fifty-five to fifty-six.

40. L. Priest, "Doctors Are Told to Warn Patients of Faulty Tests," *Globe and Mail,* 19 Mar. 2001, A1.

41. B. Kapusta, telephone interview, 6 Mar. 2001.

42. Priest, "Doctors Are Told to Warn Patients."

43. A.G. Walker, "Nova Scotia's X-Rays About 30 Years Too Old," *Medical Post,* 6 Mar. 2001, A1.

44. P. Malpass, "The Doctor Is In (In Trouble, That Is)," *Vancouver Sun,* 12 Oct. 2000, A17.

45. Kapusta, telephone interview.

46. D. Hitchlock, telephone interview, 14 Mar. 2001.

47. The overwhelming majority of these machines are located in acute care hospitals. Only provincial governments — not individual doctors — make the decision to purchase and operate them. Often the hospital administrators have limited influence. Any real authority to effect change lies with politicians and bureaucrats.

48. K. Pole, "High-Tech Assessment Body Tries to Keep Up," *Medical Post,* 6 Feb. 2001, 1.

FIVE DECADES OF OBSERVATIONS

J. Edwin Coffey

Canadian perspectives on health care are often voiced in our newspapers and on radio talk shows and television programs. Most of the evaluation is done by journalists or policy analysts. Occasionally, we hear from lawyers and politicians. Almost never, however, do we hear from physicians. In this essay, Dr. J. Edwin Coffey reflects on his career and medicare in a narrative that encompasses over fifty years.

Coffey opens with a simple declaration: "During my career, which started in general practice and later was spent as a specialist, I have had the opportunity of serving in various medical, hospital, educational, and political positions. As this experience spanned the years both before and after the profound political transformation of our health system, I have been invited to share some personal observations . . . If the following interpretations and recommendations convince our political class to apply the necessary remedies, so much the better for patients and their physicians."

Coffey begins his chronicle with his medical school days, experienced in the years shortly after World War II. He describes the mood as follows: "Except for the 1947 implementation of government-run hospital insurance in Saskatchewan, there was no indication that socialist and monopolistic health legislation would soon change the environment of the whole Canadian health care system." He goes on to describe his first practice in pre-medicare days, when he worked in Northern Quebec as a family doctor. Through anecdotes, he relates both the growing politicization of health delivery (the local hospital was built with assistance from the federal government's hospital grants program, reflecting as much political favour as absolute need) and the presence of charity work to assist the poorest citizens.

He then describes his years engaged in specialty training at Johns Hopkins and his return to Canada as the debate over national health insurance was heating up. He details the Hall Commission's work and its impact. He describes the early health care debates and his quiet approval.

The enthusiasm waned, however, as Canada in general, and Quebec in particular, opted for more and more intrusion into medical practice. The ability of physicians to extra-bill or work outside the government system was constrained. What started as an attempt to help the country's poorest citizens quickly became a major experiment in socialized medicine. Coffey describes his reservations: "I can remember trying to treat patients — many of them bleeding — in the ER in the middle of the night with no nurses available to prepare them for examination. I used to tell the medical students who were assigned to our service that they were seeing an example of Third World medicine."

He closes with a blunt assessment of Canada's medicare: "Canada's current experiment with publicly funded provincial health insurance monopolies, combined with the prohibition of alternative private health insurance and private medical and hospital services, has failed." Coffey proposes instead a move toward more individual choice and competition.

Over the past forty years, federal and provincial governments have introduced profound statutory changes in the way medical and hospital services are financed, insured, and governed in Canada. The publicly funded health insurance scheme enacted by these changes, known as "medicare," provides universal health insurance for all Canadians. There is, however, no guarantee that insured Canadians can find diagnostic equipment and treatment facilities that are up-to-date, or services that are readily accessible.

During my career, which started in general practice and later was spent as a specialist, I have had the opportunity of serving in various medical, hospital, educational, and political positions. As this experience spanned the years both before and after the profound political transformation of our health system, I have been invited to share some personal observations on this period of upheaval and offer some recommendations for the future.

The aim of Canada's current health system debate should be to develop a better understanding of the origins of our health system's decline, so we can direct our remedies to the causes rather than the symptoms. If the following interpretations and recommendations convince our political class to apply the necessary remedies, so much the better for patients and their physicians.

Med School Days

Back in the mid-1940s, when many of us entered university as premedical students, World War II was just beginning to wind down. Nevertheless, we were required to join the Canadian Officers' Training Corps (COTC) to become future officers, should the war be prolonged. We participated in army training on campus during the academic year and attended military camp during the summer. The war ended before we reached the age for active duty.

Later, as the real veterans of the war demobilized, many joined us in the medical school programs at the universities. In the late 1940s, roughly one-half of our first year medical class at McGill was composed of Canadian and American war veterans. They were slightly older and more mature than the nonveterans, and highly motivated to achieve a successful career in medicine.

Except for the 1947 implementation of government-run hospital insurance in Saskatchewan, there was no indication that socialist and monopolistic health legislation would soon change the environment of the whole Canadian health care system. None of us seemed particularly worried that politicians could adversely affect our professional careers and our ability to provide care to patients. Today politicians speak of medicare as an integral part of the Canadian identity. Back in those days, however, the notion of government-run health care would have been ridiculed.

In 1948, the federal government initiated a program to match the provinces' new health spending; much of the program was targeted at the construction of hospitals and it created a virtual hospital building boom across the country. Any federal or provincial politician worth his or her salt saw to it that the constituency would see a new hospital go up nearby.

General Practice Before Medicare

In the mid-1950s, after an internship and a year of training in pediatrics, I undertook a three-year stint as a general practitioner in a northern Quebec mining town, 565 kilometres northwest of Montreal. The town had recently benefited from the federal health grants and had built a lovely new hospital, to be run by a religious congregation of nurses. The new hospital, with its dedicated team of nursing sisters, had been one of the factors that attracted me to the area.

As this was the premedicare era, the mine employees were covered by their employer for services provided by the company doctor. They had private group hospital insurance for their families and many had medical insurance as well. Those with low incomes or who were unemployed had provincial assistance for medical and hospital costs.

I had no illusions of gaining immediate wealth from my practice, given that our office fees ranged from $2.50 to $3.75 and a hospital obstetrical delivery fee ranged from $25 to $50, and those fees were only charged if a patient could afford it or had insurance. We charged neither clergy, nurses, medical colleagues or any of their families, nor families who were obviously in poor financial health: it was considered a privilege to provide medical care for these people.

I soon discovered that those with the fewest financial resources often had the most generous hearts. For instance, I recall one young couple who was having a very rough time financially when I assisted the wife through her first labour and delivery. I delivered another baby for a poor family that already had six or seven young children. I received a call one evening from a distraught mother with a feverish and convulsing child at home. I remember that house call in particular because it came in the middle of a frigid January night. The temperature had plunged to 43 degrees below zero (Fahrenheit); the transmission oil in my Ford was so stiff that I could not shift the vehicle out of low gear, and the car's plastic seat cover split when I sat down. Later these families showed their gratitude with a delicious tourtière, a fruitbread, and a freshly cut spruce tree brought to my family's door at Christmas.

Specialty Training: Following Osler to Baltimore

After three and a half years of general practice, in the same year that Parliament enacted the universal hospital insurance program, I started four and a half years of specialty training in the United States. My first taste of high-quality American medicine came in Seattle during a short stint of residency training in surgery at the Virginia Mason Hospital, a private not-for-profit institution attached to and staffed by specialists from the Mason Clinic, often referred to as the "Mayo Clinic" of the American Northwest.

The physicians at this medical and hospital centre were first-rate. Consequently, the facility attracted many of the best graduates from American medical schools who were eager to complete their specialty training there. The clinic's reputation on the West Coast resulted in a large volume of referred patients from as far away as Alaska. Here, they received consultations with their specialists and the necessary diagnostic and treatment services under one roof. The Mason Clinic was a model of how a private specialty clinic attached to a hospital could provide efficient services of the highest quality. Most patients were covered by private insurance sponsored by their employers. Occupied with my career in Montreal many years later, I would look back to this time with envy and regret, knowing that an institution like the Virginia Mason Hospital-Clinic would never be permitted to develop in Canada.

The next stage of my specialty training began in the summer of 1958 in Baltimore. There, at the Johns Hopkins Hospital, I had the privilege to spend four years working under renowned authorities such as Eastman and TeLinde, authors of the world's two leading textbooks on obstetrics and operative gynecology at the time. I soon discovered that my McGill and Montreal General Hospital background was a key that opened many opportunities at Hopkins. Sir William Osler had gone on from McGill and Montreal General to become the founding professor of medicine at Johns Hopkins Medical School and Hospital when those facilities opened in 1889. Osler had forged a link of respect between McGill and Hopkins, a mutual respect that still exists. I benefited enormously from the legacy of generations of physicians and scientists from these two famous medical institutions, which were built, endowed, and maintained largely by the private sector to cater to the world and serve the public.

Making a Career Choice: Canada or the U.S.?

When I reached the final year of residency at Hopkins, the time came for me to make one of the toughest decisions of my career. Traditionally, the head of the department would ask a final-year resident about his or her future career plans and would make sure these ambitions were fulfilled. In my case, the decision came down to whether I would forge my career in Canada or the United States, and at which medical centre. I had always thought of returning to Montreal, but the opportunities available all over the U.S. gave me food for thought. On a family visit to Montreal that year

I talked to the department chief at McGill and Montreal General Hospital. The mood was so positive that I soon decided to return to the university and hospital where my early roots had been established.

Having just returned to Montreal in the early 1960s, and looking forward to a new career in Canada, I had some concerns upon learning about the medico-political trends that were surfacing in Saskatchewan. A physician colleague from Hopkins had just begun his career at the University of Saskatchewan medical faculty when the introduction of socialized medicine led to a doctors' strike. He and his family were threatened and his car was shot at with nail guns. As a highly trained specialist and teacher, he was not interested in stunting his career in a province where the medical and hospital systems had become so politicized. He quickly returned to the U.S. and spent the rest of his career there.

A Specialist in Montreal Before Medicare

Establishing a new practice in the heart of Montreal and undertaking some teaching duties occupied most of my time in the mid-1960s. I was fortunate to have a chief of service at Montreal General who invited me to use his downtown office during periods when he was busy at the hospital. He had a marvellous suite of antique rooms in the Old Sherbrooke Street Apartments, one of the first apartment buildings to have been built in Montreal. Its red brick facade was preserved as a heritage structure and now forms part of the south section of the Montreal Museum of Fine Arts. It was in the heart of the famous Golden Square Mile, named in the late 1800s when it was estimated that 60 percent of Canada's wealth was owned by those residing in the beautiful stone and brick homes within that square mile on the lower slopes of Mount Royal. Much of this private wealth found its way, through philanthropy, to nearby McGill University and its teaching hospitals located on the slopes.

It was not long before we moved into the new Seaforth Medical Building as part owners with the other physicians and dentists who had financed its construction through equity and bank loans. This building housed radiology, laboratory, and pharmacy facilities, along with most of the city's medical and surgical specialists and some general practitioners. The hospital was within a five-minute aerobic walk up the hill. Although my revenue barely paid the rent the first year, I was optimistic about the future. I was vaguely aware of a Royal Commission on Health Services that had been appointed by Parliament in 1961 and expected it would recommend some necessary changes in the health care system, and I had no need to worry.

Although I was quite naïve about political matters at that time, it soon became apparent that Canada was in the midst of a major debate over the future financing of medical services. The physicians' interests were represented by the Canadian Medical Association (CMA), which had proposed that voluntary medical insurance be used — like the private insurance programs already in place — and that government subsidies should be available for those unable to pay the premiums. On the other hand, the labour unions demanded that physicians be put on salary and that medical services become a public service.

The Hall Commission

In 1964, the Royal Commission on Health Services, headed by Justice Emmett Hall of Saskatchewan, reported to Parliament. The Commission had consulted health care's major stakeholders, including the CMA, and had criss-crossed the country to listen to various groups.

The Hall Commission's first recommendation was that a Health Charter, which it had already drafted, be accepted as an objective of national policy for Canada. The Charter advised that a comprehensive, universal health services program for the Canadian people be

- implemented in accordance with Canada's evolving constitutional arrangements;
- based upon freedom of choice, and upon free and self-governing professions;
- financed through prepayment arrangements;
- accomplished through full cooperation of the general public, health professions, voluntary agencies, political parties, and governments (federal, provincial, and municipal); and
- directed toward the most effective use of the nation's health resources to attain the highest possible levels of physical and mental well-being.

At first glance the recommendations sounded reasonable, in that the government would set up a prepaid medical insurance plan financed by taxation or premiums with universal entitlement to patient coverage. There would be freedom of choice for patients and physicians, and self-governance of the medical profession. There would be cooperation among all stakeholders — including members of the voluntary sector, such as commercial and nonprofit insurers — in order to attain the highest possible levels of patient physical and mental well-being. There was no mention of socialized medicine or a ban on private health insurance and private medical services in hospitals.

Over the next two years the federal and provincial governments mulled over the Hall Commission's recommendations. They hammered out arrangements for the transfer payments from Ottawa to the provinces that would pay half the cost of a universal and comprehensive medical insurance scheme known as "medicare." By December 1966, Parliament passed the appropriate medicare legislation as the Medical Care Insurance Act; it received the unanimous support of all federal parties. The federal politicians and their advisors had ignored the advice of the CMA, which was to build on the already expanding private health insurance sector and subsidize those who needed assistance with premiums.

In 1967, Canada took a breather and celebrated Expo with Montrealers, who hosted the world on beautiful and largely man-made islands in the middle of the mighty St. Lawrence. At this time, several provinces had their own assortment of private medical and hospital insurance plans and some were reluctant to convert to a publicly administered plan. However, with the Medical Care Insurance Act finally implemented in 1968, and with the generous federal contributions dangling before individual premiers, the provinces soon fell into line. One by one they passed the necessary provincial health insurance legislation and set up new government insurance bureaucracies to run medicare. Ontario's plan began in 1969 and Quebec's took hold in November 1970.

The Quebec Experience

The implementation of medicare in Quebec, however, turned out to be a nightmare. I can remember how quickly the euphoria of Expo '67 turned into general unease as a cascade of political events became entangled with a dispute between the government and physicians over the Quebec Health Insurance Act.

Earlier in 1967, Quebec's Castonguay Report had recommended major organizational changes in the delivery of health and hospital services and, as the Hall Commission had done for Canada, it prepared the way for Quebec's medicare insurance experiment.

Claude Castonguay, who cochaired the Quebec Health Commission, was soon asked to join the Liberal government as health minister. In that capacity his tasks involved

- crafting the necessary legislation to support provincial medicare and shepherding it through the National Assembly;
- dealing with the massive pressure from the left-leaning trade unions through the debates over the proposed Quebec Health Insurance Act (particularly the sections concerning (1) insurance entitlements of patients and physicians who wished to completely opt out of medicare in favour of private services and (2) the right to buy alternative private medical insurance);
- coping with the withdrawal of services (except in emergencies) by the Federation of Medical Specialists in October 1970; and
- sharing the provincial cabinet's anxiety in dealing with the October Crisis of 1970, marked by high-profile political kidnappings and the murder of a Quebec cabinet minister by the FLQ terrorist organization.

I had the occasion during this period in 1970 to share an office suite with a medical colleague who was serving on the executive of the Specialists' Federation. He was very involved with the dispute over the physician opt-out clauses in the contentious Health Insurance Act. This close association and awareness of the gravity of the medicare dispute stimulated me, for the first time, to reflect on certain values that I had always taken for granted, namely, the individual freedom and right to exercise personal responsibility in matters of health care and health insurance. Suddenly I understood how easily and quickly these values could be threatened and eroded by the political process, through a simple legislative act carried out by democratically elected representatives.

The first reading of Quebec's medicare bill had an opt-out clause, whereby a medicare-insured patient who chose to be treated by an opted-out physician would be entitled to 75 percent of the normal fee benefit. The physician could bill for the balance of the fee, if desired. A further condition was that opting out would be restricted to 3 percent of the practitioners in any specialty or district.

The specialists were very unhappy and felt this condition was discriminatory and unfair. They asked why a financial penalty should be borne by both patient and practitioner, simply because a physician chose to remain in private rather than public practice. Many physicians chose to maintain their freedom and stick with the traditional and time-honoured patient-doctor contract in which the patient receives an insurance benefit from the insurer and the physician bills the patient a fee or has the option of accepting the insurance benefit as full payment. After all, the Hall Commission had stated that the universal plan it had in mind would be based on freedom of choice and the cooperation among voluntary agents, and would not be a system of socialized or state-run medicine.

The militant trade unions were accordingly incensed that physicians should be allowed to opt out of medicare and provide private medical services to patients who preferred that alternative. Their claim was that the bill perpetuated the "intolerable privileges" of the doctors.[1] These unions pushed the government to place doctors on salary and treat them like any other government employees.

When the medicare Bill appeared in the National Assembly at next reading, the 75 percent insurance benefit entitlement to patients being treated by opted-out private physicians was reduced to zero. Thus, the desire of the left-leaning trade unions was realized. A newspaper editorial of the day stated that "Quebec is faced with a medicare act that the specialists describe, with justice, as a scheme to conscript them as salaried civil servants."

After the brief specialists' strike, Quebec medicare took hold in November 1970. Physicians and patients began to experience the advantages and disadvantages of the socialized medical insurance monopoly that augmented their existing socialized hospital insurance plan (which included a supplementary semiprivate and private hospital accommodation option). One thing was certain: if the medicare insurance experiment failed to live up to its promises of adequate financing of the health care system, there would be no parallel private health system alternative to pick up the pieces. The elimination of a private care option had been a unique and radical element in Quebec's medicare legislation, one that would be copied by other provinces and later reflected in the Canada Health Act.

The Federation of Medical Specialists and the Federation of General Practitioners were named in the Quebec Health Insurance Act to represent their respective professional groups through the negotiation of a fee schedule and the terms and conditions of medical practice and remuneration. The public fees negotiated for the specialists were considerably lower than the premedicare private fees. There was no allowance for experience and all specialists received the same fee, regardless of outstanding individual skills or experience. This practice was discouraging to those who had already invested, or were about to invest, in years of specialty training only to find that mediocrity — not excellence — was rewarded.

The Early Days of Medicare

During the first ten years of medicare, the negotiated (but essentially government-set) fees were so low that most physicians had to increase their daily caseload in order to pay overhead costs and meet the financial needs of a self-employed professional. This type of treadmill medical practice had a tendency to motivate physicians to shy away from complicated cases and concentrate instead on younger and relatively healthy patients who consumed less time. Many specialists found themselves penalized, and even harassed, by inspectors of the medicare board for providing services of higher quality than the provincial average. Discouraged, these doctors moved away to Ontario or the U.S. where their higher standards of care were welcomed.

As early as the 1970s, tardy and inadequate payments from the Quebec hospital insurance board to the hospitals forced a reduction in hospital staff and in operating room availability. These reductions were early symptoms of the deterioration yet to come in Canada's medical and hospital system. Some physicians resorted to balance-billing or user fees (even in provinces where this kind of action was illegal) to boost medicare fees to a normal level of compensation. This practice was of particular concern to the federal health minister, who appointed Justice Emmett Hall to evaluate the system that had developed since his 1964 Royal Commission proposals.

The Canada Health Act

Justice Hall recommended that the government deal with the problem by using the original Quebec weapon: the prohibition of extra-billing and user fees. He also called for compulsory arbitration proceedings to settle stalemated fee disputes between the provinces and the provincial medical associations or federations. His recommendations were incorporated into the 1984 Canada Health Act. This legislation spelled out more clearly the terms and conditions of federal contributions to provincial medicare insurance plans. If the provinces allowed extra-billing or user fees for government-insured medical, hospital, or diagnostic services, an equivalent amount of federal funds would be held back from the offending province.

In 1984, as secretary of the Quebec Medical Association (QMA), I accompanied the president to Ottawa to present the Association's views on the Canada Health Act to the Parliamentary Health Committee that was studying the bill before its passage. We were critical of the neglect by both levels of government in honouring their financial commitment to adequately fund the medicare insurance monopoly established in Quebec. Considering the health care issues that have plagued Canada in recent years, it is interesting to read some of our comments from the 1984 presentation:

> . . . our province is presently going through a crisis in health care funding. It was created by the provincial government's inability to allocate adequate resources to our hospitals in order to run them effectively and to provide quality care for patients . . . When our hospitals ask for financial aid they are told to cut back services, to centralize, to rationalize . . . These measures have already been utilized, yet we are still forced to cut more patient services . . .

> During the past 13 years, our doctors in Quebec have seen their schedule of medicare fees move steadily downward in comparison with their colleagues in other provinces until now, we are at the bottom . . . hundreds of our best trained and experienced specialists have left to relocate where their skills are rewarded . . . many who have remained are pressured into supermarket-style medicine — a little bit for everyone but quality for few. That is what the state has deemed for its citizens under Quebec medicare.

> . . . the attempt (by the proposed Canada Health Act) to force provinces to outlaw extra-billing and user fees by financial penalties, merely gives a federal stamp of approval to the punitive Quebec legislation of 1970, which made balance-billing illegal, a provision that Quebec physicians still find repugnant.[2]

The Long Decline

Now, eighteen years later in 2002, the above statements still apply. The ban on extra-billing and on private medical services is still in force. Recruiting top specialists and family physicians to the urban centres in Quebec is very difficult. Waiting times for many specialized services are disgraceful and unsafe. Emergency rooms continue to be overwhelmed.

Provincial governments continue to appoint commissions to study the symptoms of medicare's decline, but no one dares to study, or is even asked to study, the root causes of the disabled system.

I can remember trying to treat patients — many of them bleeding — in the ER in the middle of the night with no nurses available to prepare them for examination. I used to tell the medical students who were assigned to our service that they were seeing an example of Third World medicine. Such impoverishment of the medical and hospital system was predictable in light of worldwide experience with centrally planned and controlled systems of socialized medicine. This precedent was something that Canadian politicians failed to understand and over the years I have seen my worst suspicions confirmed. Looking at health care today, I see that

- many Canadians are forced to wait for or forego care, or are forced to travel to the U.S. for care at their own or at the government's expense;[3]
- restrictive medicare legislation dulls the initiative and enterprise of all health care service providers and particularly undermines the morale of physicians; and
- most of Canada's medical and hospital decision-making is politicized.

A few years before Justice Emmett Hall passed away, I had the opportunity to lunch with him in Montreal at a conference. I asked him what he thought, in view of his Royal Commission's silence on the banning of private alternative health insurance, about the current Quebec prohibition. He said his only concern was that patients have universal access to reasonable medical services regardless of financial means, and that he was not worried if people wished to buy private insurance of their own accord. I concluded from this exchange that politicians and their advisors had inserted the ban on private insurance and private medical services into health legislation for their own reasons.

Through the 1990s to the Present

The 1990s saw more evidence of central economic planning and social engineering as provincial governments cut back on admissions to medical schools; politicians' advisors declared a surplus of physicians in Canada and claimed doctors were partly responsible for rising costs. Patients were certainly not aware of a surplus as they waited for appointments. Medical associations were not aware of a surplus as they saw their numbers dwindle. Now, years after reducing the number of Canadian medical graduates, the country faces a severe shortage of both general practitioners and specialists.

The failure of Canada's provincial medicare insurance monopolies to provide accessible and high-quality medical and hospital services has come to a head over the past few years.[4] Simply closing acute care hospitals, as was attempted in Montreal, does nothing to improve access or quality and, in the process, produces severe inconvenience to and overcrowding of remaining hospitals. Pumping more money into the present system will bring some temporary relief, but there is no reason to believe that it will solve the deep structural problems.

Canada's publicly funded and provincially administered health system experiments have been carried into the new millennium on life support, and public surveys support this observation.[5] In Quebec, as in the other provinces and territories, the weight of evidence points to a serious decline in the provision of medical and hospital services furnished by these experimental health systems.[6] Surveys indicate not only a loss of public confidence in the current models of provincial health care, but paint a dubious prognosis for health care's future.[7]

Conclusion

Canada's current experiment with publicly funded provincial health insurance monopolies, combined with the prohibition of alternative private health insurance and private medical and hospital services, has failed. The experiment was founded on a utopian political and economic doctrine that has failed the world over to satisfy the political, economic, and moral expectations of citizens.[8]

The Canadian medicare experiment should undergo fundamental changes and substantial rebuilding. This statement is reinforced in recent surveys conducted by the Harvard School of Public Health.[9] Coercive health legislation that protects government monopoly and prevents private competition should be rescinded. More promising alternative arrangements for health care and health insurance should be pursued "outside the box" and without the restrictive provisions of current health legislation.

An alternative to the present single-choice medicare scheme was published by the Montreal Economic Institute (www.iedm.org) in September 2000.[10] In this study, Dr. Chaoulli and I propose a pluralistic approach to health care financing and delivery in Canada. It is a concept of health care with quality, access, and choice for all Canadians, one that will accommodate a broad range of economic and political attitudes.

While retaining universality, it would expand consumer choices for public and private financing and delivery of medical and hospital services (in line with successful European experiments). It would harness incentives such as refundable tax credits with medical savings account-type plans. This alternative encourages greater personal responsibility in health matters and, at the same time, subsidizes low-income individuals, thereby enhancing their health care choices.[11]

NOTES

1. Michel Roy, "Front Commun des Grandes Centrales Syndicales Contre le Projet de loi de l'Assurance-Maladie," *Le Devoir*, 30 June 1970, 1.
2. Dr. Marcien Fournier and Dr. J. Edwin Coffey, "Quebec Medical Association Brief," *Minutes of Proceedings and Evidence of the Standing Committee on Health, Welfare and Social Security Respecting Bill C-3, Canada Health Act* (Ottawa: House of Commons, 1984): 52–65.
3. Sean Gordon and Aaron Derfel, "Cancer Patients May be Sent to U.S.," *Gazette* [Montreal], 15 May 1999, A5.
4. See John K. Inglehart, "Revisiting the Canadian Health Care System," *New England Journal of Medicine* 342 (29 June 2000): 2007–12.
5. Angus Reid Group Poll, "71% Agree Ontario Health System Currently in Crisis," *Globe and Mail*, 17 Jan. 2000, A2.
6. "System on Life Support," *Gazette* [Montreal], 27 Nov. 1999, B6.
7. K. Donelan et al., "The Cost of Healthy System Change: Public Discontent in Five Nations," *Health Affairs* 18.3 (1999): 207–16.
8. Chiaki Nishiyama and Kurt R. Leube, *The Essence of Hayek* (Stanford: Hoover Institution Press, 1984), 123.
9. See K. Donelan et al.
10. J. Edwin Coffey and Jacques Chaoulli, *Universal Private Choice: A Concept of Health Care with Quality, Access and Choice for All Canadians* (Montreal: Montreal Economic Institute, 2000).
11. See David Gratzer's essay in this volume for more on medical savings accounts.

PUBLIC SYSTEM, STATE SECRET

David Zitner and Brian Lee Crowley

Making medicare work better in the future is the objective of every provincial government. But how well is medicare working *now*? While politicians are quick to answer this question in a positive way, do we really know how accountable and effective the system is? Saskatchewan's Commission on Medicare, headed by former Deputy Minister Kenneth Fyke, recently concluded that Canada's health care system "pays for the activity and is indifferent to the result." In this essay, Dr. David Zitner and Dr. Brian Lee Crowley investigate medicare's relationship to health information, as well as its transparency and accountability.

Zitner and Crowley consider some fundamental questions and reveal the unsettling answers. For example, "How extensive is the waiting list problem? No province can answer this question with reliable data on the appropriateness of waiting times. Nor can any province provide accurate information for an even more basic question: How many people are waiting?" Despite the inability of medicare's administrators to answer these questions, Zitner and Crowley note the impressive information tracking performed in other sectors of the economy. Medicare, however, remains a black box.

And the problem isn't just confined to the big picture, waiting times, and access. "For the most part, information sharing among family doctors, laboratories, diagnostic facilities, allied health professionals, and specialists operates at a level that people living in the days of the Pony Express would recognize: pieces of paper are mailed." That such primitive technology is used despite our awesome ability to instantly transfer data across the globe is incredible. This information gap, as Zitner and Crowley call it, means that proper data is not collected and is therefore not available. As a result, poor medical decisions are often made and there is a limited ability to reduce medical error.

The present framework leads these two authors to question why there is an information gap at all. Their conclusion is that medicare functions like an unregulated monopoly, creating a topsy-turvy world. Spending increases are viewed solely as cost increases (even if they are allotted to proven pharmaceuticals and treatments). Waiting lists are used to ration care (even if that action means patients suffer and eventually require even more costly care). Basic regulations are absent (even if the government is careful to regulate other aspects of the economy). Indeed, the very purpose of medicare — to provide for people with catastrophic illness — is thwarted. The health care system serves people with minor illnesses well, but not those who require extensive and expensive treatment.

Zitner and Crowley conclude that real medicare reform will address the present monopoly structure by introducing competition and refocusing the government's role.

1. Introduction

[B]ringing more and better evidence to bear on decisions is crucial whether by providers or by patients or managers or policy makers. Evidence offers the prospect of improving the quality of health care. That is why we are committed to closing many of the gaps that now exist in the information relating to medicine, as well as improving its quality and the use to which it is put, including through working towards a countrywide health information system. We must develop reliable, complete and objective information upon which to make judgments and upon which to make policy.

—Allan Rock, speech to the Canadian Medical Association, August 1997

In relation to the Canada Health Act, I observed that Health Canada does not have the information it needs to effectively monitor and report on compliance. So, . . . it is clear that better quality information is required.

—Auditor General of Canada Denis Desautels,
private communication to the authors, August 2000

Through the effective use of information and communications technology and the appropriate sharing of information, the fragmentation of services among health care and related sectors will be resolved and replaced with a "seamless" continuum of care within and across all services. However, major new investments will be required in information systems to support community providers.

—from the Provincial/Territorial Deputy Ministers' paper, "Understanding Canada's Health Care Costs," August 2000

Every day, the evidence becomes clearer that the health care Canadians receive is of declining quality. We spend roughly $75 billion every year on this health care, an amount projected to rise by roughly 5 to 7 percent annually. Politicians promise ceaselessly to "fix" the system, in part by introducing greater accountability for service and performance.

Much lip service has been paid to the need to improve information and accountability, but little has changed even though it was almost a decade ago that the deputy ministers of health first agreed to publish waiting times and health outcome data.[1] Politicians and their senior officials still lack even the most basic information. It is thus impossible to evaluate the quality or timeliness of the care that Canadians receive — or to properly reform our health care system.

Limited information. Modest transparency. Poor accountability. These problems are always present in an unregulated monopoly. Unfortunately, Canada's medicare system has evolved into just that. The governments that finance our health care also manage, operate, and regulate it, creating a fundamental conflict of interest. In many ways, administrators have an incentive *not* to collect and release critical information.

In this essay, we look at the information gap and its root cause. We also examine information systems in other sectors of the economy and draw important lessons for achieving meaningful health care reform in Canada.

2. Impetus for Change

What evidence is there that Canadians are not getting the health care they need and deserve?

Only 20 percent of Canadians report having confidence in the health care system, and slightly more than 50 percent say that the medical care they and their family personally received in the last year [1999] was very good or excellent.[2] A 1999 Angus Reid survey reported that over 70 percent of Canadians believe that the overall quality of care today is much worse or somewhat worse than five years ago.[3]

The public's perception appears justified when you consider the following:

- ER overcrowding is widespread and frequent.
- Seven provincial governments, including Ontario's, have been sending cancer patients to the United States.
- Though none of the measures of waiting times for treatment are satisfactory (a subject to which we shall return), the data is troubling. A raft of studies[4] looking at access to care concludes that there is "a protracted and growing wait for health services."[5]
- In 2000, an international study suggested that Canadian physicians are more worried than their international counterparts about waiting times for medical treatment.[6]

Politicians, too, appear concerned. The federal minister of health recently commented that "The health industry needs better information on what's working and what isn't. We all have heard the stories of waiting lists and the aunt who couldn't get the hip replacement for 18 months and the shortages of facilities and the difficulty getting access to diagnostic equipment."[7]

3. The Information Gap

How extensive is the waiting list problem? No province can answer this question with reliable data on the appropriateness of waiting lists. Nor can any province provide accurate information for an even more basic question: How many people are waiting?

Despite large expenditures on health information, no Canadian jurisdiction routinely collects the proper information. The largest single expenditure in provincial health budgets is for hospital care, and yet no hospital in the country can give the community it serves a meaningful account of how many people get better. (We know that the health system provides good results for many people, of course, which is a justification for our private and public expenditures.)

Canadians deserve, however, hard evidence that the tens of billions being invested on their behalf are being well-spent to achieve appropriate health outcomes. Moreover, they want assurances that providers are tracking and linking activities and results in order to reduce medical error, redundant tests, and ineffectual clinical practices.

Consider the following brief list of questions to which, in any jurisdiction in Canada, no one can provide satisfactory answers:

- How many people have difficulty finding a family doctor?
- Who got better, who got worse, and whose health status remained unchanged as the result of contact with the health care system?
- Is the cost for improving health status higher or lower in rural areas than in urban centres?
- Who is waiting for care?
- How long have they waited?
- Who waited too long, given their current health status?
- Which specialties have unacceptably long waiting periods?

These basic questions deserve answers — not for academic interest, but for the policy-makers who need guidance when they are deciding how to marshal their resources. Nevertheless, major decisions are made despite the lack of information. Closing and amalgamating hospitals; removing (and subsequently adding) hospital beds; allocating specific resources; and graduating certain numbers and types of physicians from our medical colleges — all these major decisions are made without the benefit of timely, useful, and clear information. And while the usual rational criteria are invoked to justify these decisions, the harsh reality is that they are based on anecdotes, "gut feeling," or political considerations.

The situation is well-described by Healnet (Health Evidence Application and Linkage Network):

> Many bad decisions about health care are made every day in Canada because decision-makers lack the right information, at the right time, and in the right place. These bad decisions can cost the country millions of dollars and rob Canadians of the health care they need and deserve. Decisions that are made about the health system — like funding for diagnosis and treatment of many diseases — are only as good as the information on which they are based.[8]

There is no justification for this information gap. The means to gather and interpret needed data exist. Contrast the black box of health care with the privately managed segments of the economy. For instance, bed management tools — something almost unheard of in the Canadian hospital sector — are commonly used in the hotel industry. And when it comes to information gathering, the private sector has no difficulty tracking waiting times for cars, bank tellers, flights, groceries, or anything else.

It is possible to argue that health care delivery is more complicated than, say, flight arrival times. But in reality, the complexity is readily handled. The data gathering program Caretrak identifies on a daily basis who should be in a hospital and who is more appropriately cared for in another setting, and yet the program is not widely used in any province — not even in the Maritimes where it was developed. And Caretrak isn't the sole choice in this area. CONTINUUM is a similar product. Both produce information in real time and encourage appropriate use of resources.

Despite the availability of such tools, health administrators in Canada continue to use diagnostic labels to measure resource use. With diagnostic labels, patients are grouped into crude (and ultimately useless) categories. A pneumonia patient on IV antibiotics in the ICU of a hospital has the same disease classification as a relatively healthy patient in the community who is taking oral drugs. You don't need a medical degree to see the difference in health status between these two people, but with diagnostic labels, health administrators are effectively blind to the distinction.

Other jurisdictions offer useful lessons about the use of information technology. In Pennsylvania, for example, all health care institutions are required to use Medigroups, a computer program that tracks patient characteristics and treatment. Medigroups also predicts mortality risks, providing a crude but effective performance measure.[9] Pennsylvanian health organizations are required to participate in assessments involving their total number of cases, the number of cases in each category, the risk-adjusted length of hospital stay, the risk-adjusted mortality, and the average charges per case. Pennsylvania collects and reviews information, not just about diagnoses, but also about illness severity. The state also posts information about organization performance on the Internet for all to see. Institutions with excessive costs or high death rates have a very strong and public incentive to make improvements.

Contrast this kind of accountability with our information gathering techniques. Consider that if a patient is discharged from a Canadian hospital but dies the next day, it is recorded as a successful health care encounter.

The Information Gap on Health Care's Front Lines

Unfortunately, even those who recognize that Canada suffers from a dearth of information about the health care system tend to think only in terms of the big picture, waiting times and access. These elements represent only one small part of the information system's inadequacy.

Quality and timely information is vital for proper diagnosis and treatment. But what sort of information support does your doctor's office have? It has been estimated that the average physician must be able to marshal

hundreds of thousands of pieces of information in order to properly diagnose and treat the range of illnesses that patients will present in normal
practice. A good family doctor will thus have an impressive memory. But
doctors aren't psychics — they need test results and consults. For the most
part, information sharing among family doctors, laboratories, diagnostic
facilities, allied health professionals, and specialists operates at a level that
people living in the days of the Pony Express would recognize: pieces of
paper are mailed. Even in major Canadian teaching hospitals, data is often
stored on loose-leaf sheets in souped up three-ring binders.

Consider the awesome amount of data moved and manipulated in every
day life: you can fly to Bangkok and withdraw money from an ATM; you
can look up your stock portfolio on the Internet and make trades; you can
pay all your bills over the phone. But in the health care system, there is
little e-technology and a lot of post office.

Clinicians gather important information about patient health and they
scrawl notes onto charts. Written and stored on paper, this data is not available to support care elsewhere and it cannot be used to gather systematic
information about the results of care. The collection, analysis, and distribution of information derived at the point of care clearly leads to improved
knowledge and outcomes, as has been documented, for example, with pediatric cancer patients.[10]

There is another major advantage to employing information technology
at the point of care: it helps reduce medical error. Prompting systems, for
instance, remind clinicians of patient allergies, body weight, and prescribed
medications, allowing them to avoid drug side effects and interactions.
Ironically, one of the major developers of prompting software used by
American clinics and hospitals is a Toronto company.

Medical errors impose a great economic cost. And with the recognition
that medical errors lead to more fatalities than motor vehicle accidents,
breast cancer, or acquired immune deficiency syndrome (AIDS), major
attempts are being made to reduce such mistakes south of the border.[11]

Canada has not followed the lead of the United States in putting resources
into encouraging error reduction, even though there is every reason to
believe that our situation is at least as bad as it is in the United States. As is
the case with better patient tracking in hospitals, the necessary technologies exist to bring Canadian primary care into the twenty-first century —
or at least into the twentieth century.[12] (A study in the *Canadian Medical
Association Journal* reported that only 16 percent of adult patients with

hypertension received drug treatment and had normal blood pressure. Most people have annual contact with a health professional at a walk-in clinic, a family doctor's office, or an ER. We wonder if more people would be appropriately treated for high blood pressure if information were readily available, thus sparing thousands from the disability and death caused by heart attacks and strokes.[13])

Poor-quality health care and the information gaps that exist within the health care system are not separate and unrelated issues, but are instead intimately linked.

4. Our Diagnosis: An Unregulated Monopoly

Wal-Mart uses satellite technology to update data in its central computers every time a purchase is made in any North American store. Managers use this information to determine which products sell and where. Banks use data mining techniques to predict which customers are likely to default on loans. Supermarkets use these techniques to predict buying patterns in a particular store. In health care, these tools would be useful as part of routine health system monitoring in order to learn which activities benefit the public, which waste money, and which are harmful. But Canadian health care is a monopoly — there is little incentive to fret about customer needs. Actually, it's much worse than that — health care is an *unregulated* monopoly, devoid of any performance requirements.

This lack of appropriate information tools and technical infrastructure would not be acceptable in any industry where consumers have a choice among competing suppliers. A company, 50 percent of whose consumers are dissatisfied, would likely not survive for long. Not surprisingly, private sector organizations work feverishly to avoid such a scenario, obsessively collecting information pertaining to their performance.

Consumer-driven companies regularly survey their customers to learn if they are satisfied. Yet how many Canadians have been called and asked if their health improved following medical care or if they waited too long in an ER?

In a competitive environment, it's recognized that the right knowledge at the right time in the right hands is not only power, but also the key to success. There is a common exception to this rule, however. Monopolies, whether public or private, are notoriously indifferent to the satisfaction of their customers: by definition, a monopoly's customers are unable to choose another supplier.

Canadians instinctively understand these truths about monopoly behaviour. Consider the concern expressed at the near-monopolistic power that Air Canada has acquired. The public knows that as the sole national airline, the company has a unilateral ability to determine flight schedules and seat sales.

Yet as much as Canadians clearly mistrust monopolies in general, they seem oblivious to the fact that their public health care system is a classic monopoly. Thus, we cannot properly evaluate, for example, the sources of Canadians' satisfaction or dissatisfaction. As a virtually unregulated monopoly, administrators do not collect proper information about the strengths and weaknesses of health delivery.

As an unregulated monopoly, health care has many problems in addition to the information gap. A few of these problems are discussed below.

Goals and Incentives

The private sector attempts to gain market share and attract and retain customers. It values innovations that improve efficiency and foster the development of new products and services, thus increasing market share.

As a tax-financed monopoly, health care's funding isn't directly derived from satisfied consumers, but from political negotiations instead. Consequently, spending increases are viewed as cost increases, regardless of whether certain expenditures may create more value for patients. For example, provincial governments fret about rising drug costs and create obstacles for physicians prescribing expensive but effective pharmaceuticals, encouraging them to prescribe cheaper alternatives instead — even if these alternatives have a greater likelihood of producing side effects.

Complicating this picture further are the various disincentives for providers. Doctors who attract a sicker and more complex patient population are penalized by the fee-for-service structure because such patients take longer to see. Under block funding, hospitals have little incentive to innovate for or to consider the needs of the communities they serve.

Queue Management

Businesses in a competitive industry gain an advantage by providing timely service. Most managers recognize that a fifteen-minute wait at the local supermarket's checkout line is unacceptable. Some banks even promise cash awards to customers if they wait too long in the queue.

Since the health care monopoly is unconcerned by dissatisfied consumers, administrators ration through waiting in the name of cost containment. Evidence, however, suggests that longer waiting times may drive up costs because health deteriorates while a patient remains unseen (leading to prolonged disability, repeat physician visits, and more expensive and technical interventions).

Regulation

The private sector is subject to government regulation. For example, governments regulate the production, quality, and safety of meat products. They set hygiene and freshness standards for raw meat, as well as guidelines for the use of chemicals. Governments require that meticulous records relating to these issues be kept. Additionally, labour regulations govern working conditions. And, to ensure transparency, manufacturers are required to disclose ingredients and best-before dates.

But while businesses face heavy regulations, government-provided health care delivery does not. Governments don't set standards for appropriate waiting times and pertinent information regarding access to care isn't disclosed to the public.

In summary, an unregulated monopoly occurs when a particular group captures a market, has no competitors, and is able to assess its own performance without the need to comply with a set of external regulations. Where Canadian health care is concerned, these conditions have been met because the government

- defines what constitutes "medically necessary services";
- pays for all such services provided;
- prevents Canadians, by law and regulation, from obtaining such services outside government channels;
- administers and governs care, either directly or indirectly; and
- assumes responsibility for defining, collecting, and reviewing information regarding its own performance.

5. The Information Black Hole:
CIHI and Health Care Accountability

Canada *appears* to have made a national commitment to collect appropriate information by establishing the Canadian Institute for Health Information

(CIHI). Indeed, CIHI is the lynch pin of the federal-provincial efforts to increase accountability.

CIHI is funded by the federal government to the tune of $95 million, and has a national mandate that includes identifying information needs and priorities and collecting, processing, and maintaining data for various health databases and registries.

According to the CIHI Web site, "[T]hrough the pursuit of these primary functions, CIHI helps its many clients to make sound health decisions based on quality health information. Stakeholders include ministries of health, health care facilities, health-related organizations and associations, the research community, private sector and the general public."[14] CIHI has substantial influence, and determines what information health organizations will collect and use.

In addition to federal funding, each province contributes to CIHI. Most Canadian hospitals contribute data to the CIHI discharge abstract database, at significant cost; for a 400–500-bed hospital, the cost for abstracting discharges ranges between $1 million and $1.5 million.

Unfortunately, this huge investment in information is largely ineffective. Health record reviewers record diagnoses, but collect no information about a patient's comfort and level of functionality before and after treatment, reason for admission, or waiting time. Diagnostic labelling is ineffective at best, dangerous at worst.

But this inefficiency doesn't prevent CIHI from analyzing the data collected.[15] Based on this flawed data set, CIHI sends hospitals a report that includes average length of stay for a particular diagnosis.[16] Without adjustments for severity of illness or other variables, comparisons among health organizations are misleading. Hospitals have no way of knowing if the lengths of patients' stays are too long or too short. Despite detailed reviews of each page of a discharged patient's record, health record reviewers don't collect the most pertinent information.

6. Implications of an Unregulated Health Care Monopoly

Canadians often hear that they have the "best health care system in the world." While flag-waving may be rewarding, it does little to address basic questions about timeliness and quality of care.

As with any other forms of monopoly, the Canadian health care system cuts itself off from vital information for two reasons. First, a monopoly by its nature generates no feedback from customers who have the option of switching to an alternate supplier. Second, because information about our health care system's performance may be used to assess the performance of medicare's administrators, it is not in the interest of these administrators to collect it — they are in a conflict of interest.

On this latter point, consider the Ontario government's handling of emergency room overcrowding. In fall 2000, ministry officials decided to stop releasing information on hospital redirects (in effect, the number of emergency rooms not receiving patients due to overcrowding). Such data, after all, reflected poorly on the government. Administrators, in other words, deliberately undermined transparency for political purposes.

The Powerless Consumer

In a competitive environment, consumers "vote with their feet." They did so in the 1970s when they abandoned North American cars for cheaper and better Japanese imports. Over the years, they have switched from slide rules to calculators and from regular mail to e-mail.

But in a monopoly — even a regulated one — the relative power of consumers and suppliers is completely reversed. Before the advent of competition in the telephone industry, a dissatisfied customer faced the massive indifference of a bureaucracy that could literally take its business for granted. This kind of behaviour was common, even though politicians (who are answerable to voters) had a theoretical hand on the tiller through regulatory agencies.

Like their cousins in the monopoly family, administrators of the Canadian health care system suffer no direct consequences as a result of poor customer service. Other than the ineffective channels for registering complaints with politicians, letters to the editor, and calls to open line shows, dissatisfied consumers have little power. A powerless consumer must face excessive waiting times and suffer medical errors. While the information is spotty, the studies we cited at the beginning of this essay give a clear indication that these problems are real and growing.

The other phenomenon at work here is the emergence of various forms of black and grey markets for health care provisions, ranging from the in-house medical services offered by some employers to the public sector agencies (such as Workers' Compensation Boards) with favoured access to public health care resources. These practices almost always facilitate queue jumping.[17]

A Paradox: Unresponsive Monopoly, Massive Change

It has been said that the best monopoly rent is a quiet life.[18] Recent studies show that monopoly managers normally have quieter lives than those in highly competitive fields.[19] But Canadian health care is in turmoil and the administrators have a tumultuous life. Medicare is constantly restructured and reorganized. Unfortunately, without changing the fundamental ways in which care is provided and without measuring the outcomes, the reforms seem to be exercises in pushing rope.

Those responsible for the health care system are caught between two painful realities. On the one hand, the public's angst is palpable — health care is a major issue in federal and provincial elections, often to the detriment of governing parties. On the other hand, efforts to reduce spending or to make resources go further are really little more than guesses about what might work, since so little information is available.

The Insurance Function

Another consequence of the health care monopoly is the corruption of the basic insurance function. All Canadians pay for health insurance through taxation, allowing them to share the financial cost of risk. Insurance is most beneficial when it protects against a risk for which an individual could not normally pay (e.g., the cost of a heart transplant). It is less beneficial when it pays the cost of an inexpensive risk, such as a cold or a flu. (In fact, the cost per person of insuring all Nova Scotians for a heart transplant is virtually the same as insuring for minor respiratory illnesses.[20]) Increasingly, however, administrators balk at expensive, but proven, treatments.

In the case of new cancer treatment, the latest pharmaceuticals (such as visudyne for macular degeneration), and cutting-edge diagnostic tests, Canadian governments reduce their expenses by limiting service. Yet it is doubtful that individuals would make that kind of choice if they themselves were purchasing health insurance. If economies must be made, it makes more sense to pay a small amount to insure fully for catastrophic events, but to buy more limited coverage for minor complaints (consider that people buy home insurance with a low deductible, but rarely insure for plumbing repairs).

But the administrators of a politicized monopoly like medicare see things differently. They have every reason to reduce the frequency of expensive procedures and drug use (exactly the items that would require insurance) because these items affect few people and carry a heavy price tag.

7. Improving Quality and Accountability

In Canada, provincial governments are the monopoly. Provincial governments not only pay for necessary care, but also govern, administer, and evaluate the services they themselves provide. Self-regulation never works. But there are two ways to curb this monopoly's power: (1) introduce competition and (2) refocus the government's role.[21]

To introduce competition while maintaining the valuable aspects of a public health insurance scheme, it is essential to unbundle the payment, administration, delivery, and evaluation functions.

Governments should set strict performance requirements (such as appropriate waiting times for high-quality care) and then tender out services. To win contracts, bidders would compete, thus encouraging cost savings. On its most superficial level, this result could be accomplished with an internal market; Sweden, the United Kingdom, and New Zealand operate with this kind of system. In Sweden, for example, this approach resulted in a significant increase in cost savings, efficiency, and patient satisfaction.[22] (This structure can even be taken a step further through medical savings accounts, as described in David Gratzer's essay in this volume.) Additionally, an independent evaluator would be responsible for regularly reporting to the public about access and outcomes.[23]

Governments should ensure that no one goes without quality medical services, which is a vibrant but limited role. As has been described in this essay, the basic problem with health care today stems from the overarching role of government. As a result, Canadians pay billions of dollars into an unregulated monopoly.

Canadians often express their surprise at the fact that medicare no longer works well. The real surprise is that it ever did.

NOTES

1. *When Less is Better* (Ottawa: Conference of the Federal/Provincial/Territorial Deputy Ministers of Health, 1994).
2. N.P. Roos, "The Disconnect Between the Data and the Headlines," *Canadian Medical Association Journal* 163.4 (2000): 411–12 and Canadian Institute for Health Information, *Health Care in Canada 2000: A First Annual Report* (Ottawa: CIHI, 2001).

3. Angus Reid Poll Group, Poll 53 in "Public Policy Focus: Canadians' Perspectives on Their Health-Care System and 'Social Union,'" *Angus Reid Report*, Jan./Feb. 1999, 18.
4. For a brief survey of these studies on access and waiting times, see David Gratzer, *Code Blue: Reviving Canada's Health Care System* (Toronto: ECW Press, 1999).
5. M. Zelder and G. Wilson, *Waiting Your Turn: Hospital Waiting Lists in Canada*, 10th ed. (Vancouver: The Fraser Institute, 2000).
6. Barbara Sibbald, "Canada's MDs Most Pessimistic in 5-Country Survey," *Canadian Medical Association Journal* 163.11 (2000): 1496.
7. Tom Spears, "The Waiting Game: The Elderly Suffer Most as Canadians Across the Country Find Themselves Waiting Longer for Hospital Treatment," *Ottawa Citizen*, 5 Oct. 1999, D9.
8. Healnet (Health Evidence Application and Linkage Network), "Gap in Health Information Management Puts Canadians at Risk," press release, Hamilton, ON, 15 Oct. 1999.
9. For examples of the detailed evaluations this software makes possible (including data appropriately adjusted for the severity of individual patient illnesses), see www.phc4.org/reports/hospitals.htm.
10. J.V. Simone and J. Jane Lyons, "Cancer Survival in Children Compared to Adults: A Superior System of Cancer Care," *Health Affairs* 19.6 (2000): 9–20 and Committee on Quality Health Care in America, *Crossing the Quality Chasm: A New Health System for the 21st Century* (Washington: Institute of Medicine, 2001).
11. L.T. Kohn, J.M. Corrigan, and M.S. Donaldson, eds., *To Err is Human: Building a Safer Health System* (Washington: National Academy Press, 2000).
12. B. Crowley, D. Zitner, and N. Faraday-Smith, *Operating in the Dark: The Gathering Crisis in Canada's Public Health Care System* (Halifax: Atlantic Institute for Market Studies, 1999) and D. Zitner, G. Paterson, and D. Fay, "Methods to Identify Pertinent and Superfluous Activity," in *Health Decision Support Systems*, J. Tan, ed. (Gaithersburg: Aspen Publishers. Inc., 1998).
13. M.G. Myers, "Compliance in Hypertension: Why Don't Patients Take Their Pills?" *Canadian Medical Association Journal* 160 (1999): 64–65.
14. CIHI Web site, www.cihi.ca/weare/weare.htm, 16 Dec. 2000.
15. CIHI, *Health Care in Canada 2000*.
16. The rankings by CIHI constitute a form of league table. Those hospitals at the top of the league maintain shorter length of stays for a particular set of ICD codes or diagnoses compared with the hospitals at the bottom of the league, which have longer stays. However, in the absence of appropriate adjustments for severity or statements about the benefits of care, it is not possible to know if a length of stay is appropriate in a particular circumstance. Restructuring or changing health services organizations based on the current league table methodologies is "equally likely to be beneficial, harmful, or irrelevant." See CIHI, *Health Care in Canada 2000* and J. Parry et al. "Annual League Tables of Mortality in Neonatal Intensive Care Units: Longitudinal Study," *BMJ* 316 (27 June 2000): 1931–935.
17. Lisa Priest, "Hospital Reviewed Own MRI Practices," *Globe and Mail*, 21 Dec. 2000, A7 and Dave Frances, "For Rent: Medical Services," *Times & Transcript*, 20 Dec. 2000, A1.
18. J. Hicks, "Annual Survey of Economic Theory: The Theory of Monopoly," *Econometrica* 3 (Jan. 1935): 1–20.

19. C.E. Fee and C.J. Hadlock, "Management Turnover and Product Market Competition: Empirical Evidence from the U.S. Newspaper Industry," *The Journal of Business* 73.2 (2000): 205–43.

20. Crowley et al., *Operating in the Dark*.

21. "Tackling Monopolies," *The Economist*, 7 Feb. 1998, 80.

22. See Johan Hjertqvist, "The Purchaser-Provider Split: Swedish Health Care Reform — From Public Monopolies to Market Services," www.fcpp.org.

23. We have limited faith in the current movement toward report cards, as health organizations are reporting on their own performance and are generally saying that the care they provide is excellent.

PART 3

LOOKING AHEAD

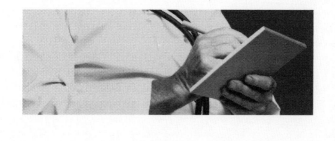

POPULATION MATTERS: DEMOGRAPHICS AND HEALTH CARE IN CANADA

David Baxter

Much health care analysis tends to focus on the here and now. We read about emergency room overcrowding, nursing shortages, and other immediate problems. But a major challenge to Canada's health care system lies in an underappreciated issue: our aging population. Consider that during medicare's golden age (the mid-1970s), the average Canadian was 19 years old. In 1998, the typical person was 36. Based on demographic forecasts (not adjusting for migration), by 2030 the average age could be 68. In this essay, David Baxter examines the relationship between demographics and health care spending in Canada.

To understand the future better, Baxter begins by looking at spending patterns over the past two decades. Baxter explores private and public spending, birth and mortality rates, and expenditures by age group. Noting the six-fold increase in provincial government spending between 1975 and 1998, Baxter explains the escalation and concludes that for the most part, aging played a modest role in the spending increases (14¢ of every new dollar).

But aging will have a bigger impact in the future. Baxter observes that the demographic wedge — the 43% of Canada's population currently in the 31–60 age group (often and erroneously termed the baby boom generation) — will move from being tax contributors to heavy health care users.

Looking solely at aging, the country's current demographics will increase the required average per person contribution from the 20–64 age group by an average of 1.46% per year — triple the rate of increase experienced over the 1975–98 period. And such a projection is by its nature conservative, as aging is just one cost pressure on medicare. Baxter also calculates that with increased immigration and reduced emigration, taxpayers will still face roughly double the annual rate of increase seen since the 1970s.

In other words, without any change in spending patterns — that is, without any change in today's health care system — Baxter suggests that we must anticipate a major increase in the financial requirements needed to support provincial government spending.

Baxter's conclusion? "Demographics will not determine either the quality or the characteristics of health care in Canada in the future; these will be determined by how we respond to the pressures that demographic change — along with technological, social, economic, and environmental change — will bring. What we cannot deny is that change will occur."

1. Introduction

Demographic analysis — the study of factors that determine the size and composition of populations — is much overrated: puffery, not reality, underlies the slogan "Demographics Explain Two-Thirds of Everything." Pseudo-demographic projections of everything from stock market booms to housing market meltdowns have been so wildly wrong that they have raised questions about the very validity of demography as an area of study. Critics now refer to demographics using terms such as "voodoographics" and "doomography." This is unfortunate because demographic analysis, when correctly and judiciously applied, is both a useful and a powerful tool.

There is great potential for demographic analysis to contribute to the ongoing discussion of change in Canada's health and medical care (hereafter referred to as health care) system. Demographics are strongly influenced by health care, particularly with respect to changes in death rates and birth rates. More significantly, health care is influenced by demographics. The patterns of causes underlying both illness and mortality are highly correlated with age, as are the rates of utilization of doctor, hospital, and care services; medical laboratories; and pharmacists. As a result, significant changes in the age composition of Canada's population will have noticeable effects on the level of health care demand.

In this essay, I examine the historic role of demographic change in determining the level of health care spending in Canada, and the extent to which it may affect such spending in the future. I begin with an examination of the age-specific pattern of provincial government health spending in Canada, followed by an examination of the current demographic composition of Canada's population and of the forces that shaped it. These two elements of health care demand are then used to measure the extent to which demographic change contributed to the more than sixfold increase in provincial government health care spending in Canada between 1975 and 1998. Finally, these demographic and spending patterns are used to project the magnitude of increase in provincial health spending that will occur in the future if demographics alone determine health care spending.

2. Provincial Government Health Care Spending in Canada

The Role of Provincial Governments

There are a number of reasons for selecting provincial government spending as the example in a discussion of demographics and health care. Some of these reasons are prosaic; one is pragmatic. The pragmatic reason is that the most current and comprehensive data on the demographic pattern of health spending available is for the provincial government sector: the 1998 data on per capita provincial government spending by age group published by the Canadian Institute for Health Information (CIHI) enables both analysis and projection of the effects of demographic change on provincial government health spending.[1] No data on corresponding currency or comprehensiveness are available for either private spending or spending by the rest of the public sector. Given the currency of the provincial data, 1998 is used as the reference year for this analysis of the relationship between demographics and provincial government health care spending.

On the prosaic side, one reason for considering provincial government health care spending is that it is the single largest component of health care spending in Canada. Its 1998 expenditure of $54.10 billion accounted for 64% of the total $83.96 billion spent on health in 1998, and 92% of the total $58.85 billion spent on public sector health care (see Figure 1).[2] These figures compare with 30% private, 4% direct federal, 1.2% social service agency, and 0.8% municipality spending on health care.

Between 1975 and 1998, provincial government spending on health care increased by 521%, from $8.71 billion in 1975 to $54.10 billion in 1998. While this $45.39 billion was the largest absolute increase in sectoral spending on health care, it represented the smallest percentage increase. For instance, federal direct spending increased by 676% (from $0.40 billion to $3.09 billion) and private spending increased by 766% (from $2.90 billion to $25.11

FIGURE 1

Health Spending in Canada by Sector, 1975 and 1998

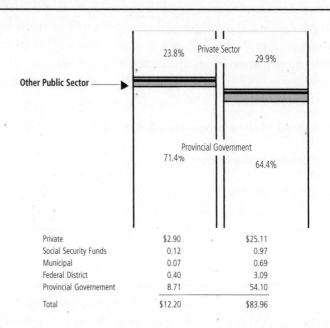

	1975	1998
Private	$2.90	$25.11
Social Security Funds	0.12	0.97
Municipal	0.07	0.69
Federal District	0.40	3.09
Provincial Governement	8.71	54.10
Total	$12.20	$83.96

billion). As a result of its relatively slow growth rate over this period, the provincial government share of total health spending declined by 7.0%, from 71.4% in 1975 to 64.4% in 1998, while each of the other sectors' shares increased. The largest share increase occurred in the private sector; its spending increased from 23.8% of all health spending in 1975 to 29.9% in 1998.

A second reason for focusing on the relationship between demographics and provincial government health care spending is that there is evidence to indicate that provincial spending will experience greater pressures for expenditures as a result of future demographic change than will the other sectors. A 1994 Health Canada report provided spending estimates for each major sector by major age group and sex for the 1980–94 period.[3] According to these data, 49% of all provincial government spending was on people aged 65 and older, compared with only 34% of other government spending and 14% of private spending (see Figure 2).[4]

Private spending has the largest proportionate share in each of the under 65 age groups, a factor largely explained by the fact that dental and vision care services are largely private expenditures incurred before one

FIGURE 2

Age Distribution of Sectoral Health Spending in Canada, 1994

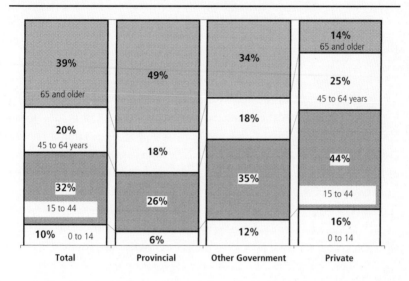

reaches age 65. In 1998, private spending accounted for 94% of all payment for dental services, 91% of all payment for vision care services, 68% of all payment for services of other nonphysician health professionals, and 69% of the prescription and nonprescription drugs purchased in Canada. The public sector accounted for 99% of the spending on physician services and 91% of the spending on hospital operation and services, expenditures that are largely incurred after we reach age 65.

The 1994 data, viewed from a different perspective, show that provincial government spending accounted for 84% of all spending in the 65 and older age group, but only 59% in the 45–64, 55% in the 15–44, and 44% in the 0–14 age groups. Private spending accounted for only 11% of all spending in the 65 and older age group, compared with its 35% share in the 45–64, 39% in the 15–44, and 49% in the 0–14 age groups.

A final reason for selecting provincial governments is that their role in health care extends far beyond spending; it is provincial governments who establish the fiscal and regulatory environment within which health care operates. Provincial governments are responsible for public health, ranging from water quality standards to inoculation programs. They are responsible for licensing, contracting, and regulating health care delivery; educating health care practitioners; and establishing employment standards.

Provincial governments' response to the shifting pressures that demographic and other changes will bring to health care in the future will largely determine the characteristics and quality of health care in Canada.

The Life Cycle of Provincial Government Health Spending

The reason that provincial government health spending is particularly sensitive to changes in the age distribution is immediately obvious from Figure 3, which shows the estimated average amount spent by provincial governments in 1998 on health care per person in each age group.[5] The life cycle of health spending starts at a relatively high level during the first year of life — an average of $4,812 per person — and then declines steeply, first to an average of $774 in the 1–4 age group, and then to the lowest average spending of $581 per person in the 5–9 age group. From this age group on, the average amount spent each year per person increases to reach its highest value of $21,312 for each person in the 90 and older age groups. This age-specific pattern provides the key to the exploration of both the historical and future impacts of demographic change on provincial health spending in Canada.

From age group 1–4 to age group 50–54, the average amount spent per person each year on health care is below the overall average spending of

FIGURE 3

**Provincial Government Health Care Spending
by Age Group in Canada, 1998**

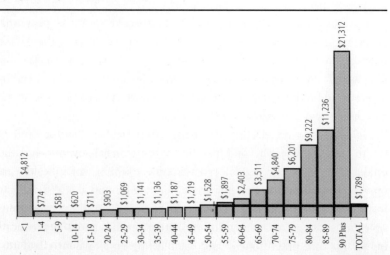

$1,789 per capita; for every age group 55 and older, spending per capita is above the average. All other things being equal, any demographic change that increases the percentage of the population that is in older age groups will mean that provincial health care spending will increase faster than the population, and faster than the spending in the rest of the public sector and in the private sector.

On its own, Figure 3 may create too strong an impression of the age sensitivity in provincial government health spending. While the highest spending occurs in the oldest age groups, not all of the population reaches those age groups; at today's life expectancies, only 59% born will reach the average life expectancy of 79 years, and only 23% will reach the highest spending 90-plus age groups. Current life expectancies and expenditure patterns combined mean that provincial governments spend an average of $196,182 per person on health care during that person's lifetime: 12% is spent before age 25, 14% is spent between the ages of 25 and 50, 30% is spent between the ages of 50 and 75, and 44% is spent after the age of 75. The bottom line: Given projected demographic changes for Canada — even adjusting for life expectancy — provincial governments will experience a dramatic increase in health spending if current expenditure patterns prevail in the future.

3. The History and Characteristics of
Canada's Current Population

Births are the major determinant of both the size and age composition of Canada's population; of the 28.5 million people counted in the 1996 Census, 83% were born in Canada.[6] As a result, the historical pattern of births, as shown in Figure 4, largely explains the shape of the current age profile of Canada's population, as depicted in Figure 5.[7]

While Canada's population increased during the 1911–36 period, the annual number of births remained relatively constant in the 240,000 births per year range. As a result, the number of births per 1,000 people declined steadily from its century high of 31.9 births per 1,000 in 1915 to what was then a record low of 20.1 per 1,000 in 1936 and half of the 40 births per 1,000 recorded at the time of Confederation. The year 1937 marked the turning point in the direction of both the birth rate and the annual number of births. From 1937, the birth rate climbed to a plateau in the range of 28 births per 1,000 from 1948 to 1958. Then, following a decline in the num-

FIGURE 4

Annual Number of Live Births in Canada, 1911 to 1998

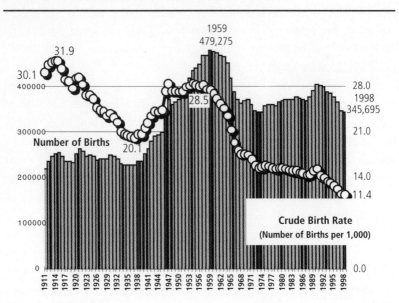

ber of births due to a growing (and aging) population, it fell relatively steadily to reach its historical low of 11.4 births per 1,000 in 1998.

The annual number of births also increased dramatically after 1937, taking a big jump in 1946 to reach Canada's record of 479,275 births in 1959. The number of births then started to decline, slowly at first, and then steeply after 1963 until 1978, when the rate of declined slowed. In 1973, the trend reversed and the number of births increased to 400,000 by 1990 before declining again to reach 345,695 in 1998, a number only slightly above that of 1946.

Turn Figure 4 (annual number of births) on its side and you have, essentially, the 1998 age profile of Canada's population shown in Figure 5.[8] There are a number of ways to characterize this age profile. One is to impose upon it the concept of a generation, traditionally a 20-year age group that is assumed to represent the age difference between parents (one generation) and their children (the next generation). This concept is the basis for the currently popular invention of a "postwar baby boom generation," representing those born during the period of a relatively high number of annual births from 1946 to 1965. Aged 33–52 in 1998, these 9,682,800 "baby

FIGURE 5

Age Profile of Canada's Population, 1998

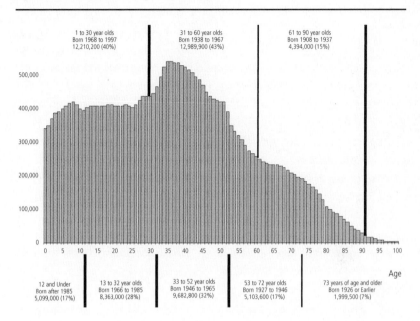

boomers" accounted for 32% of the country's 30,248,000-person population that year. Corresponding to the record number of births that occurred between 1959 and 1963, the most typical "baby boomers" would be the 2,684,800 Canadians (9% of the population) aged 35–39 in 1998. If the "postwar baby boom" is indeed a generation, then the 5,103,600 people (17% of the population) born between 1927 and 1945 and aged 53–72 in 1998 compose that group, and the 8,363,000 people (28% of the population) born between 1966 and 1985 and aged 13–32 in 1998 compose a third generation.

While perhaps convenient, there are a number of drawbacks to this generational imposition. First, the median age of a woman who gives birth in Canada is 28, and hence there is no demographic basis for a 20-year generation span. Nor is there a strong functional basis. Perhaps there would have been in the distant past when cultural and social change occurred very slowly, and people shared values and behaviours with those born between 15 and 20 years before or after them. But today, no one would seriously argue that a 52-year-old is similar enough to a 33-year-old to be placed in that group rather than one composed of 53- or 54-year-olds.

Third, and of more concern, is that the imposition of arbitrary generations, particularly ones delimited by external factors (e.g., the end of a
war), obscures both the shape and implications of the age profile. For
example, the current vogue of focusing on the *postwar* baby boom generation, with predictions of future booms and busts triggered by its aging,
obscures the fact that Canada's boom in births, and hence the major factor
that determined the shape of its age profile, began in 1938, well before the
postwar period. This means that the rapid increase in health care spending
that, all other things equal, will accompany the aging of the people born
during this boom will begin much sooner than would be anticipated using
generational analysis.

A second way of looking at an age profile is from the perspective of
demography, specifically the historical pattern of births. Note that the 1998
age profile begins to widen noticeably at age 60, which corresponds to the
increase in the number of births in Canada in 1938. It continues to widen,
with a considerable step outward at age 52 (corresponding to the jump in
births in 1946), to reach its widest point at ages 35–39 (corresponding to
the peak in births between 1959 and 1963). From age 35, the profile shrinks
significantly (as did the annual number of births between 1963 and 1968)
until it reaches a relatively constant width at age 30. The age profile of the
population is relatively constant between the ages of 30 and 9, as were the
number of births from 1968 to 1990, albeit with a slight bulge in the 7–9
age group to match the slight bulge in births from 1988 to 1991. The post-
1990 decline in the annual number of births is shown in the shrinking of
the age profile in the 8 years of age and under population, with fewer
people of each younger age, corresponding to the decline in births between
1991 and 1998. In 1998, there were fewer people under the age of 1 in Canada
than there were people of every other age up to 52; that is, up to the number of people born in 1946, corresponding to the similar number of births
in the two years.

The historic pattern of births and the age profile are essentially, but not
exactly, the same. The match is not perfect because war (e.g., the Korean
War), increasing life expectancy, and changing levels of immigration (e.g.,
the higher-than-average levels in 1951–52, 1966–67, 1973–75, and post-1989)
and emigration (e.g., the recent brain drain) have all contributed nuances
to the shape of the age profile. Nonetheless, the pattern is clear: if Canada's
age profile is considered directly rather than through the artificial lens of
generations, the issues of an aging population and health care are immedi-

ate, not a decade or more in the future. (In fact, as discussed in the next section, the aging of Canada's population over the past quarter century is partly, but not wholly, responsible for the current health care crisis in Canada.)

In conclusion, the boom in births in Canada between 1938 and 1967 created a demographic wedge in Canada's age profile. This wedge, the 12,959,900 persons aged 31–60 in 1998, accounted for 43% of Canada's population. The 30-year age group that precedes this wedge, the 4,394,000 persons aged 61–90, accounted for only 15% of the country's population, while the 12,210,200 persons aged 1–30 accounted for only 40%.

The wedge is poised to enter the 65-plus age group, which will swell the number of people in these high average per capita provincial health care spending age groups. The impact that the aging of this wedge will have on the demand for provincial government health spending can be both measured and predicted. Before doing so, however, it is important to consider the impact it already has had.

4. The Historical Impact of Demographic Change on Provincial Health Spending

The 521% increase in provincial government spending on health care, from $8.7 billion in 1975 to $54.1 billion in 1998, followed a pattern of steady increase from 1975 to 1992 and then remained relatively constant in the range of $49 billion until 1997, when it resumed its growth to reach $54.1 billion in 1998 (see Figure 6).[9] Other public spending also grew steadily from 1975 to 1993, and remained relatively constant in the range of $4 billion during the 1993–96 period, and then increased to $4.7 billion by 1998. By contrast, private spending increased continuously from 1975 to 1998, even during the mid-1990s, when it moved up from $19.6 billion in 1993 to $22.4 billion in 1996 and on to $25.1 billion in 1998. Figure 6 also shows the preliminary data for sectoral health spending in 1999 and 2000.

Provincial government spending is estimated to have increased by an average of 7.1% over these two years, more than twice the 1990–98 average of 3.1% per year. Spending by other public sector agencies is estimated to have increased by an average of 8.4% per year (above the 5.2% annual average for 1990–98) and private spending is estimated to have increased by 4.7% (below the 1990–98 annual average of 6.1% per year). Because of the preliminary nature of the data for 1999 and 2000, and because the data

FIGURE 6

Health Care Spending by Major Sector in Canada, 1975 to 2000

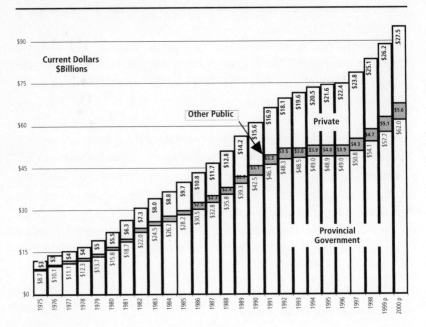

on age-specific spending is only available for 1998, the reference period for the analysis presented here will be from 1975 to 1998.

To determine the extent to which changes in Canada's population contributed to the increase in provincial government spending, it is necessary to examine each of the three factors that drive provincial spending: demographics (population growth and change), general inflation, and changes in the costs and consumption of provincially provided health care.

Population Growth and Change

To measure the share of the increase in provincial health spending over the past two and a half decades that resulted from population growth alone, it is necessary to calculate what health care spending would have been each year if the only element that changed was the number of people in Canada. In other words, the age-specific health spending pattern and the age composition of the population must be held constant. This is done by applying the 1998 age distribution percentage of Canada's population and the 1998

age-specific provincial health spending pattern to the actual population of
Canada in each year between 1975 and 1998.[10]

If provincial age-specific health care spending patterns and the age distribution of the population were the same in 1975 as they were in 1998,
with a 1975 population of 23,143,000, provincial health spending would
have been $41.4 billion dollars (see Figure 7). The only difference between
the numbers used to calculate this value and those that determined the
$54.1 billion spending in 1998 is population growth, from 23.1 million to
30.2 million. Population growth alone, therefore, was responsible for an
increase of $12.7 billion (the 31% increase from the 1975 population-based
value of $41.4 billion to the actual 1998 value of $54.1 billion) in provincial
health spending. The total growth in provincial spending between 1975 and
1998 was $45.4 billion. In this growth from $8.7 billion to $54.1 billion, 28%
was solely due to the 31% increase in the country's population.

In 1998, provincial governments spent an average of $1,789 per person
on health care; if population growth was the only factor that caused change
in health care spending, governments would have spent the same amount
per capita in 1975. The actual amount spent per capita in 1975 was $376, so
obviously factors other than population growth were the major determi-
nants of the change in provincial health spending over the 1975–98 period.

FIGURE 7

Provincial Government Health Care Spending in Canada, 1975 to 1998

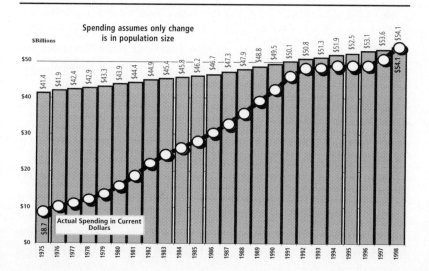

One of these factors was the aging of Canada's population that occurred between 1975 and 1998. While the aging of Canada's population is often discussed as though it is something that will only occur in the future, it has, in fact, occurred almost continuously during the past century. Part of this aging is the result of increasing life expectancies; only 5% of Canada's population in the 1900s was 65 years of age and older, compared with 7.5% in the 1950s, 10% in the early 1980s, and 12.3% in 1998. Another part of the aging has been due to the decline in the annual number of births since 1963; as soon as one year's births adds fewer people to the population than the previous year's births, the average age of the population increases.

The aging of the population between 1975 and 1998 is shown in Figure 8. Clearly observable in both the 1975 and 1998 age profiles is the demographic wedge born between 1938 and 1967. In 1975, the wedge was aged 8–37, and accounted for 52% of Canada's population and fit into one of the lowest-cost stages in the life cycle in terms of provincial government health care spending. The introduction of publicly funded, universally accessible provincial health care systems in the early 1970s could not have had a more fortuitous demographic environment.

Between 1975 and 1998, this wedge progressively aged up the population age profile, reaching progressively higher average per capita annual spending age groups along the way. In 1975, the median age of Canada's population was 27, the typical Canadian was a 19-year-old, and only 8.5% of the population was 65 years of age and older. In 1998, the median age was 36, the typical Canadian was a 36-year-old, and 12.3% of the population was 65 years of age and older. This aging has had a significant and measurable impact on the demand for provincial health spending over the past quarter century. Measuring that impact requires (1) the assumption that provincial government age-specific health spending was constant at the 1998 amount and pattern over the 1975–98 period, and (2) the application of this per capita age-specific average spending to the actual population — in terms of both size and age distribution — that resided in Canada each year. By holding spending patterns constant, demographics can be isolated as the only source of change in total provincial spending.

On the basis of this assumption, in 1975, provincial governments would have spent a total of $35.0 billion on health care (see Figure 9). With the amount and pattern of per capita spending held constant, the only factor able to cause a change from this calculated 1975 value to the $54.1 billion spent in 1998 is demographic change, which therefore accounted for a 55%

FIGURE 8

Age Profile of Canada's Population, 1975 and 1998

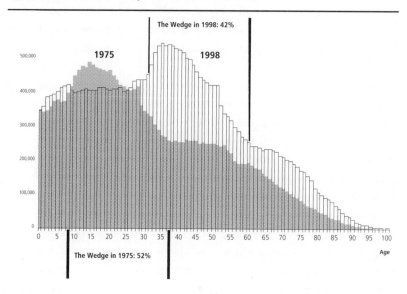

FIGURE 9

Provincial Government Health Care Spending in Canada, 1975 to 1998

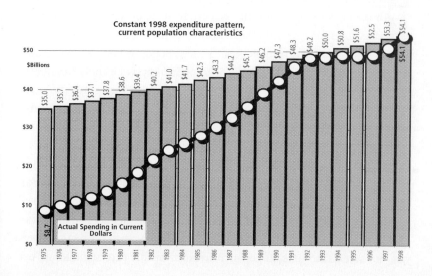

($19.1 billion) increase in health spending, and 42.2% of the total increase of $45.4 billion. Demographic change includes both population growth and changes in the age profile; population growth accounted for an increase of $12.7 billion (28% of the total increase) and the changing age composition accounted for an increase of only $6.4 billion (14.2% of the total).

The aging of Canada's population between 1975 and 1998, therefore, had a significant impact on provincial health spending, as 14.2% of the total increase in health spending in this period can be accounted for solely by the fact that 1998's population is older than 1975's. However, even when population growth is added to the impact of population change, demographics explain only 42% of the increase in provincial government health spending over the past two and a half decades.

If 1998 health spending patterns and costs prevailed, per capita provincial government health care spending would have been $1,511 in 1975; in 1998, per capita spending was $1,789. This means that there was an 18% increase in per capita provincial health care spending in Canada solely because the median age of Canada's population increased from 27 to 36 between 1975 and 1998.

Per capita spending implies a focus on recipients, but it is also important to consider spending per contributor. While there are many ways to define the contributory population for provincial health spending, the most convenient way to define it in the current context is demographically. In this case, the 20–64 population is defined as the contributory age group for our pay-as-you-go health care system. In 1998, provincial government health care spending was $2,918 per contributor (i.e., per person aged 20–64). If provincial government health care spending had remained unchanged over the 1975–98 period, spending in 1975 would only have been $2,736 per contributor. Thus, the change in the country's age profile between 1975 and 1998 resulted in only a 7% increase in per contributor expenditure. The reason the increase is so small is that the demographic wedge was in the contributory population throughout this quarter century period. In fact, between 1975 and 1984, the aging of the last of the demographic wedge into the contributory population resulted in a decline in per contributor spending to $2,702 (assuming constant age-specific spending per capita).

Actual per capita provincial government health spending in 1975 was only $376, far less than the $1,511 that it would have been if demography was the sole cause of changes in provincial health care spending. This means that the major factors in increased provincial government health spending were general inflation and changes in the amount and/or pattern of provincial average per capita age-specific health spending.

Inflation

The 1970s and 1980s were periods of very high inflation in Canada, with prices and incomes chasing each other in what at the time seemed an ever widening spiral; the basket of commodities that consumers could buy with $100 in 1975 cost $200 in 1983 and $270 in 1990.[11] The perceived consequences of this inflation were so severe that controlling inflation became, and remains, the mantra and the mission of governments and central banks. The result of their efforts has been that, over the past decade, annual inflation has been generally in the 1%–2% per year range, compared with the 10% per year range of the early 1980s.

The role of general inflation in the historical increase in provincial health care spending can be measured using current dollars, rather than the assumption of constant dollars that is implicit when using 1998 dollar amounts for provincial age-specific spending. This measurement is accomplished by converting the 1998 dollar values to their equivalent purchasing power in previous years using the Consumer Price Index for the 1975–98 period. The result is an age-specific spending pattern with exactly the same relative pattern, but expressed in current rather than constant dollars. For example, the 1998 average spending of $1,136 per person in the 35–39 age group would have involved spending only $361 per person in 1975. Using current population size and composition and 1998 spending patterns expressed in current dollars results in a 1975 provincial government health care expenditure of $11.1 billion, compared with the $35.0 billion that would have been spent using constant dollars (see Figure 10). General inflation alone, therefore, accounted for an increase of $23.9 billion in provincial health spending, contributing 52.6% of the total increase in provincial government health spending over the 1975–98 period.

Total spending in 1975 was $8.7 billion current dollars, compared with the $11.1 billion that would have been spent if general inflation and demographic change were the only factors affecting provincial government health spending. Thus, there remains $2.4 billion in increased spending (5.3% of the total) that cannot be explained by either general levels of inflation or demographic change. This remainder must be attributable to changes ultimately

FIGURE 10

Provincial Government Health Care Spending in Canada, 1975 to 1998

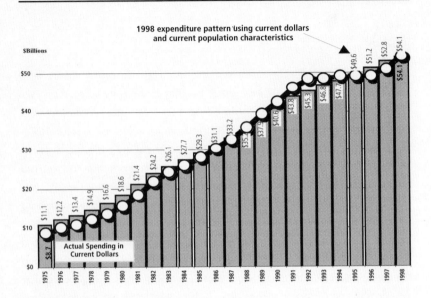

reflected in the pattern and/or the amount of age-specific provincial health care spending.

Without annual age-specific spending data for 1975 and subsequent years, it is not possible to identify the extent to which this additional growth was attributable to unique inflation in the provincial health sector (changes in prices) and to changes in the consumption of provincially provided health services (changes in use).

Two important points can be made as a conclusion to this historical analysis. The first is that general inflation was the major factor contributing to increases in provincial government health care expenditure over the 1975–98 period, accounting for 53% of the total increase. Population growth was the second most important factor, accounting for 28% of the total increase. Changes in the population's age composition (aging), while a significant factor, accounted for only 14% of the total increase. Combined, these three factors accounted for 95% of the change in provincial health spending over the period.

The second is that these factors had different impacts over different periods of time. For example, data for the 1980–94 period indicate that, of the increase in all health expenditures over this 15-year period, general inflation accounted for 42.2%, population growth for 8.4%, and changes in the population's age composition for 3.8%, while above-average price increases in the health care sector and increases in consumption of health care services accounted for 44.8%.

In this context, the period between 1993 and 1996, when provincial spending remained essentially constant at $49.0 billion (it actually declined between 1994 and 1995), is very significant. During this period, general inflation was low, but still positive; population growth was not high, but still positive; and aging, while proceeding one year at a time, still occurred. For provincial spending to remain constant during this period, there had to be reduction in provincial costs due to a fall in the prices paid by provincial governments and/or a reduction of significant magnitude in real per capita spending in one or more age groups to pull down the per capita average.

Data on inflation in both government spending and health care spending indicate there was inflation — not deflation — in health prices during this period. While it cannot be proven using available data, anecdotal evidence — ranging from increasing queues and waiting lists to growth in parallel domestic and cross-border private health care providers — suggests that per capita spending was reduced through a reduction in services rather than a decline in prices. It will be extremely useful to revisit this analysis in two years, when the results of the 1999, 2000, and 2001 increases in provincial health spending are reflected in per capita age-specific data, to see the extent to which the additional spending merely represents a "catch-up" for the 1993–96 period.

5. The Future

While of interest in its own right, the historical analysis presented in the preceding section has greater importance in providing the tools and the methodology for projecting the impact of future demographic change on provincial health spending. To make this projection, it is necessary to put aside the issues of inflation (either general or unique to the health care sector) and changes in the utilization of the health care system. This is accomplished by (1) assuming that the 1998 age-specific provincial health spending pattern remains unchanged — in both pattern and amount — in the future and (2) applying this pattern to the projected future populations of Canada. This assumption does not argue that inflation and changes in spending patterns will not occur; the assumption is merely made to keep the focus on the role of demographic change, leaving the discussion of the other topics for another place and time.

The Impact of Canada's Current Population on the Future of Health Care

One of the major topics in the debate about Canadian health care is the impact that the aging of our current population will have on future health care spending. This impact can be measured — as by definition it excludes changes in everything but demographics — by projecting the demographic future of Canada's current population, and applying current (1998) age-specific spending patterns.

In order to describe the demographic future of Canada's current population, it is necessary to use a population projection technique (traditionally called a natural increase model) that starts with the current population by age and sex composition and, using prevailing age and sex-specific mortality and birth rates, projects the population size and composition into the future. This technique differs from a standard population projection only in that it does not consider immigration and emigration. This projection shows that biology alone would lead to a long-run decline in Canada's population.

The reason for current biological factors leading to a long-run decrease in Canada's population is that the average number of children women in Canada give birth to during their lifetime is 1.7 (see Figure 11).[12] This total fertility rate is below the average of the slightly more than 2 children per woman necessary for a population to replace itself, a level that Canada has not experienced since 1970 (1.7 children do not replace 2 adults).

A second — and more important in the current context — implication of a below-replacement-level birth rate is that at this level, the average age of the population continually increases. While the 2 older people remain in the population (and given current life expectancies, they'll remain for a long time), they account for a greater share of the population than the 1.7 younger people that the birth rate adds to it.

Compounding the aging effect of a below-replacement-level birth rate is the timing of births. Throughout the past half century, the age at which women give birth has increased, effectively increasing the share of the population in the older age groups by widening the distance between the age of parents and that of their (partial) replacements. For example, in

FIGURE 11

Total Fertility Rate in Canada in 1921 to 1997
Average Number of Children Born per Woman During Her Lifetime

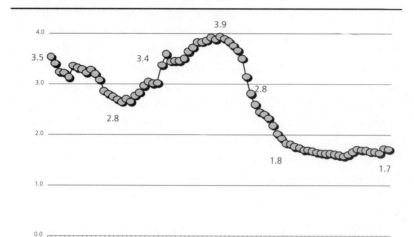

FIGURE 12

Age-Specific Fertility Rate in Canada, 1998
Percentage of Women in Age Groups Giving Birth During Year

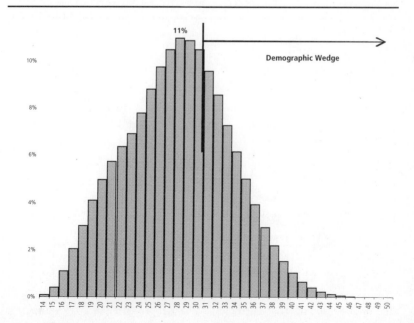

1966, the median age for women giving birth was 25, with only 30% being 30 years of age or older; in 1998, the median age was 28, with 46% being 30 or older (see Figure 12).[13]

The pattern of change in both the rate and timing of births means that, without net immigration, the annual number of births in Canada will continue to decline unless there is a dramatic change in the reproductive behaviour of Canadian females. Given trends in the availability of birth planning technology, urbanization, and labour force participation rates, such a behavioural change is unlikely. More importantly, the population of females of childbearing age is declining; the demographic wedge has essentially aged through the childbearing stage of the life cycle. In the absence of net immigration of young people, the spiral of a below-replacement-level birth rate and an aging population will combine to reduce the number of births, setting the stage for a further reduction in the number of births years into the future.

The pattern of mortality rates will also contribute to the continued aging of Canada's population in the future. At today's mortality rates, the people in the demographic wedge may have moved out of the stage in the life

FIGURE 13

Age-Specific Mortality Rate (Logarithmic Scale) in Canada, 1998
Annual Number of Deaths of Persons of Each Age per 100,000 Persons of That Age

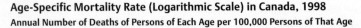

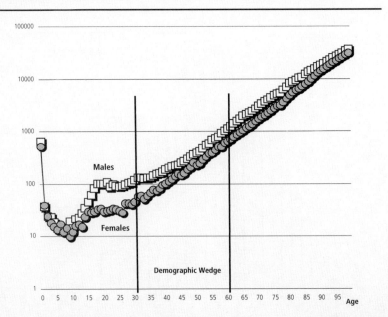

cycle where they have a high propensity to have children, but they still have a long time left to age before they reach the high mortality rate age groups (see Figure 13).[14] At current mortality rates, half of the people alive in Canada today will be alive in 45 years — and will be 45 years older.

Compounding the long life expectancies that current mortality rates represent is the changing trend in mortality rates, which have demonstrated a steady decline over the past half century (see Figure 14).[15] If this trend continues, even if at a slower pace than in the past, it will push mortality further into the future for today's population and, as a result, increase the proportion of the population in the high provincial health care spending age groups.

Ignoring the declining trends in both birth and death rates (and thereby having a slightly low estimate of the relative size of the future older population) and assuming no immigration or emigration permits projection of the demographic of Canada's current population using prevailing birth and mortality rates.[16] The result is a population relatively constant in number (declining by only 2%, from 30,248,000 in 1998 to 29,614,500 in 2030) but one that is getting rapidly and significantly older (see Figure 15).

Our long life expectancies will ensure that the demographic wedge born between 1938 and 1967 will still be apparent in the 2030 population, but it

FIGURE 14

Age Standardized Mortality Rates, Canada in 1950 to 1997
Deaths per 100,000 Persons, Standard Age Profile

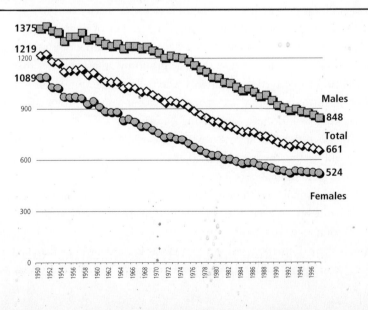

will have moved up the age profile. Considering today's mortality rates, of the 12,989,900 people aged 31–60 in 1998, 7,947,000 will be alive and between the ages of 63–92 in 2030, accounting for 27% of the 2030 population of 29,614,500 that would result from natural increase alone. Without migration, the typical person in Canada in 2030 would be a 68-year-old, 32 years older than the typical 36-year-old person of 1998.

The shift up in the age profile means that the number of people aged 52 and older will increase, with the greatest percentage increases occurring in the 65–74 age groups.

The fact that in 1998 there were fewer people of every age under age 27 than there were people between the ages of 28 and 51 means that the number of people between the ages of 32 and 51 will decline between 1998 and 2030; without migration, there are not enough younger people in Canada's population to replace the current population in the 51 and under age groups. This fact, combined with a below-replacement-level birth rate, means that the number of births to this natural increase population will decline every year in the future, continuously shrinking the number of young people and narrowing the bottom half of the age profile at the same time that aging is broadening the top half.

Natural increase alone — the future consequence of the 1998 age profile and current birth and death rates — will almost double the number of people in Canada aged 65 and older, from 3,745,200 in 1998 to 7,229,300 in 2030. For every 1 person in this age group in 1998, there will be 1.93 in 2030, which will not only be the most rapid increase of three major age groups, but the only increase (see Figure 16). The number of people aged 20–64 will increase slightly between 1998 and 2010, as the number of people aged 8–19 in 1998 who will age into this age group by 2010 is greater than the number of people aged 53–64 in 1998 who will age out of it. From 2010 on, however, this contributor age group for pay-as-you-go provincial health care systems will decline continuously, until it is 90% of its 1998 size by 2030 (from 18,542,200 in 1998 to 16,683,600 in 2030). The under 20 age group will decline the most; in 2030, there will be only 71 people for every 100 there were in 1998 (7,960,600 in 1998 to 5,701,700 in 2030).

If natural increase is the sole determinant of demographic change, than in 2030, one out of every four people in Canada will be 65 years of age or older (compared with today's one in eight). This increase in the oldest age group's share of the population, from 12.5% to 24.5%, will be matched by a decrease in the 20–64 age group's share from 61% to 56%, and in the 0–19

FIGURE 15

Canada's Population Age Profile, 1998 and 2030
Natural Increase

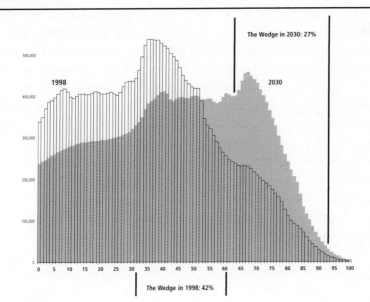

FIGURE 16

Growth of Age Groups in Canada's Population, 1998 to 2030
Natural Increase

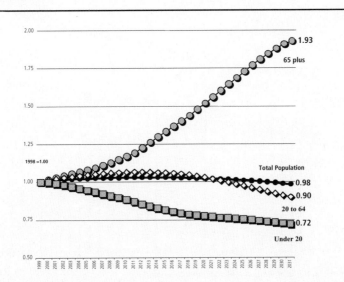

age group's share from 26% to 19%. Under natural increase conditions, this concentration of Canada's population in the oldest age group and the decline in the total size of the population will continue as long as today's long life expectancies and below-replacement-level birth rates prevail.

The implications of the aging of Canada's population resulting solely from its current demography (i.e., without migration) are dramatic. For example, if age-specific health spending patterns remain exactly as they were in 1998, with no inflation and no increases in age-specific per capita consumption of provincial health services, provincial health spending will increase from $54.1 billion to $72.7 billion between 1998 and 2030 (see Figure 17). This 34% increase will be a real (i.e., constant dollar) increase that will occur if spending patterns remain at their 1998 level.

Note that this is a conservative (i.e., low) projection; the preliminary data for 1999 and 2000 show provincial health expenditures increasing by an average of 7.1% per annum over the past two years, more than twice the 1990–98 average of 3.1% per year. These recent increases are above the rate of inflation, the rate of population growth, and rate of population aging, and hence must also involve real increases in age-specific per capita spend-

FIGURE 17

**Projected Provincial Health Spending in Canada, 1998 to 2030
Natural Increase Only**

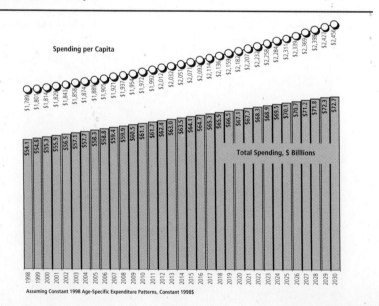

ing. As a result, the use of 1998 age-specific spending data, the most recent available, will lead to a conservative estimate of future real health spending.

As the population will be essentially constant during this period, real per capita spending will increase by a greater percentage — 38% (from $1,789 per person in 1998 to $2,456 per person in 2030). This increase, determined solely by demographic change under natural increase conditions, is more than twice the 18% increase that demographic change brought to per capita health spending in the 1975–98 period.

The growth in per capita health spending will take place at a time when the number of people in the 20–64 contributory age group is declining. The result will be that the amount that each member of the contributory population must put into the pay-as-you-go provincial health care system will increase from $2,918 in 1998 to $4,360 in 2030 (see Figure 18). Under natural increase conditions (assuming no inflation and no change in health services), the 38% growth in real provincial health spending resulting from the aging of Canada's current population will require a 50% increase in contributions. Aging of the population increased the load on the contributory population by only 7% between 1975 and 1998; the demographic

FIGURE 18

**Projected Provincial Health Spending in Canada, 1998 to 2030
Natural Increase Only**

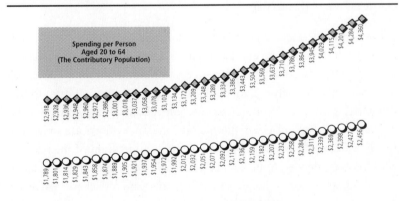

Spending per Person
Aged 20 to 64
(The Contributory Population)

Spending per Capita
(per person in the population)

Assuming Constant 1998 Age-Specific Expenditure Patterns, Constant 1998$

wedge was in — or aged into — the contributory population during this period, but had yet to reach the high health expenditure age groups. Over the next thirty years, the wedge will age out of the contributory population and into the high expenditure age groups.

It is the magnitude of the real increase on the contributory population's load in the future (based on our current health care system and our current demography) that raises concern about the ability to fund the system (that is, using 1998 age-specific spending patterns) in coming years. Considering only demographic change, provincial health spending divided by the size of the contributory population increased from a low of $2,702 per contributor in 1984 to $2,918 per contributor in 1998, which represents an annual average increase of 0.43% per year. The contingent provincial health spending liability represented by our current demographics is an increase on the contributory population's load that averages 1.26% per year, or three times the amount experienced over the past fifteen years.

Demographic analysis makes it absolutely clear that our health care system will — and must — change in response to the life cycle pattern of system utilization. Acknowledging rather than denying that change must occur is the first step in planning for it. Ready or not, the change is occurring.

The Impact of Canadian Population Trends on the Future of Health Care

For labour force reasons, Canada has historically had a policy of attempting to attract immigrants and has been, to a varying degree, successful in doing so. Discussed less often, however, is the fact that Canada also loses people to other countries (and is doing so at an increasing rate), something that is evidenced not only by anecdotes about a brain drain, but also by data. While both of these international migratory flows are small relative to the size of Canada's population, any consideration of the relationship between demographic change and health care spending in Canada must address these two issues. The natural increase model adequately describes the contingent liability for our health care system represented by our current age profile and mortality and birth rates. However, a population projection that considers immigration and emigration gives a better representation of the full demographic environment for the future of health care.

FIGURE 19

**Age Profile of Canada's International Migration
1997 to 1998 Average**

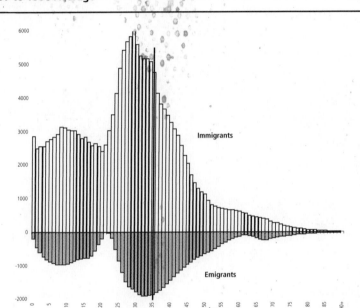

Immigration and emigration have significant demographic characteristics, as both have age profiles that are distinctly younger than the current population of Canada (see Figure 19).[17] In 1998, 48% of Canada's population was under the age of 35; in 1997 and 1998, 70% of the immigrant population and 56% of the emigrant population was under the age of 35 (see Figure 19). Immigration supplements the contribution of births to the number of · people in Canada who are younger than the demographic bulge, while emigration offsets this contribution. Simply put, all other things being equal, the lower the immigration rate and the higher the emigration rate, the faster Canada's population will age; the higher the immigration rate and the lower the emigration rate, the slower Canada's population will age.

The levels of both immigration and emigration are small relative to the number of births and deaths. Over the past decade, immigration has ranged from a high of 265,405 people (0.87% of the population) in 1993 to a low of 173,011 people (0.57% of the population) in 1999 (see Figure 20).[18] This immigration data represents half the contribution of births, which ranged from a high of 403,000 (1.5%) in 1990 to a low of 340,900 (1.1%) in

FIGURE 20

Canada's Immigration and Emigration, 1987 to 1999

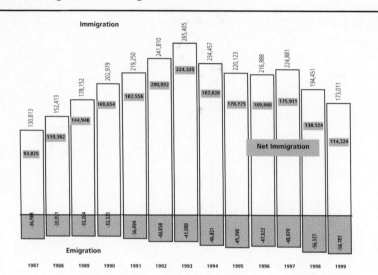

1999. While immigration generally declined over the past decade, however, emigration increased from 33,325 people (0.12% of the population) in 1990 to 58,787 (0.19% of the population) in 1999. This data compares with the increase in deaths from 192,600 (0.70%) in 1990 to 222,400 (0.73%) in 1990.

Declining immigration and increasing emigration means that net immigration (the difference between the two international migratory flows) declined by 50% over the past decade, from a net contribution of 224,325 people to Canada's population in 1993 to only 114,224 in 1999. As net immigration supplements the contribution of (a declining number of) births to the size of the younger population, this trend is of concern; if it continues, it means the relative size of the contributory population in the future will be smaller than it would be otherwise.

In projecting the level of future immigration and emigration, the federal Liberal government's policy goal of 1% immigration per year, given both the trend in immigration and the competitive environment that exists for immigrants, seems a bit optimistic.[19] It is here assumed that the immigration rate will increase to stabilize at 0.75% of the population and that the emigration rate will decrease to stabilize at 0.16% of the population. If these levels can be attained, the population of Canada will grow by 24% to 37,490,600 people in 2030. As net immigration adds not merely people, but

FIGURE 21

Canada's Population Age Profile, 1998 and 2030, 0.75% Immigration

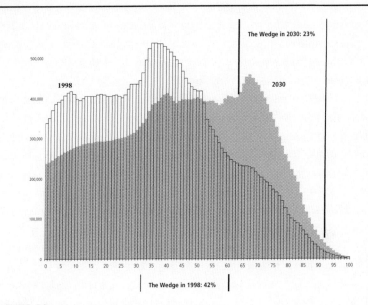

FIGURE 22

Growth of Age Groups in Canada's Population, 1998 to 2030, 0.75% Immigration

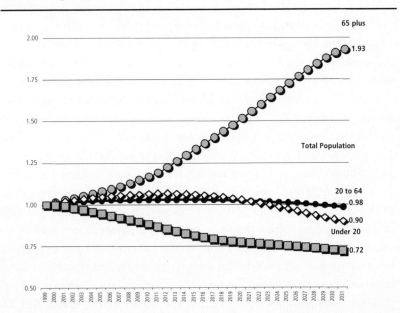

specifically young people, this projected growth will reduce — but not eliminate — the effects of our current population's aging. The demographic wedge will still be apparent in the age profile in 2030, with those aged 62–91 accounting for 24% of the population (see Figure 21). The young age profile of migrants, however, will mean that the base of the age profile will remain essentially at its current size rather than shrinking as it would without international migration.

The number of people aged 65 and older in Canada's population will still demonstrate the greatest rate of increase over the projection period, from 3,760,000 people in 1998 to 7,756,100 people in 2030 (see Figure 22). However, unlike the natural increase scenario, the number of people aged 20–64 will also increase by 18%, from 18,616,000 people in 1998 to 21,945,900 people in 2030. The under 20 age group will decline very slightly if the assumed levels of net migration can be attained, from 7,992,000 people in 1998 to 7,788,600 people in 2030.

The result will be a population that is older than it is today, but younger than it would be without migration. In 2030, one out of every five people in Canada will be 65 years of age or older, compared with today's one in eight and the one in four resulting from natural increase alone. The 65-plus age group's share of the population will increase from 12.5% to 20.7%, which will be matched by a decrease in the 20–64 age group's share from 61% to 58%, and a decrease in the 0–19 age group's share from 26% to 20.8%. If the growth pattern is followed, there will be almost the same number of people under the age of 20 in 2030 as there are people 65 years of age and older; natural increase, on the other hand, would create a situation with 25% more people aged 65-plus than people 19 and younger.

Population growth will mean an increase in health spending. If age-specific health spending patterns remain exactly as they were in 1998, with no increases in either inflation or consumption of health services, then under this scenario, provincial health spending would increase by 56%, from $54.1 billion in 1998 to $84.3 billion between 1998 and 2030 (see Figure 23). On a per capita basis, provincial health spending would increase from $1,789 per person in 1998 to $2,249 per person in 2030. This is a 26% increase, compared with the 38% increase per capita that would occur without migration. It is the fact that migration is concentrated in younger, below-average provincial health spending age groups that leads to a smaller increase in per capita spending with immigration than without it.

The situation is similar when consideration is given to the load of this

FIGURE 23

Projected Provincial Health Spending in Canada, 1998 to 2030
0.75% Immigration

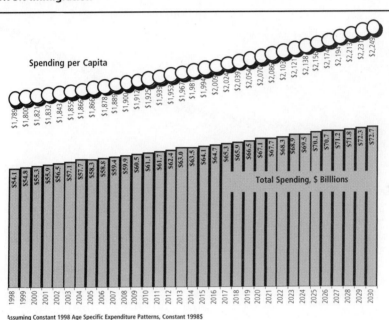

Assuming Constant 1998 Age Specific Expenditure Patterns, Constant 1998$

spending on the contributory (aged 20–64) population (see Figure 24). Under this scenario, provincial governments would go from needing to collect $2,918 from every person in the contributory population in 1998 to needing to collect $3,843 from each of them in 2030, an increase of 31% compared with a 50% increase that would occur without net immigration. On an annual average basis, this represents an increase of 0.86% per year over the next thirty-two years, twice the average increase of 0.43% experienced over the 1975–98 period, but two-thirds the 1.26% average annual increase that would occur without migration.

6. Conclusions

Population matters. The change in Canada's age profile over the 1975–98 period increased the provincial health care spending per capita contribution of the 20–64 age group from $2,736 to $2,918, an average increase of

FIGURE 24

Projected Provincial Health Spending in Canada, 1998 to 2030
0.75% Immigration

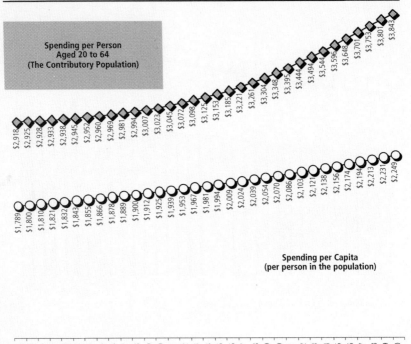

Spending per Person
Aged 20 to 64
(The Contributory Population)

Spending per Capita
(per person in the population)

Assuming Constant 1998 Age Specific Expenditure Patterns, Constant 1998$

0.43%. If Canada is able to attain immigration at a rate of 0.75% per year
and reduce emigration to a rate of 0.16% per year, the increase in the
amount required per capita from the contributory population will increase
from $2,918 to $3,843 by 2030, an average increase of 0.86% per year. Without migration, the increase will be from $2,918 to $4,360 per person in the
contributory population, an average increase of 1.26% per year.

Much — but not all — of this increase is the result of Canada's current
age profile, which has 43% of its population in the 31–60 age group poised
to enter the high per capita provincial government health care spending
age groups. This wedge is much larger than the 15% of the population currently aged 61–90 that it will replace over the next thirty years. It is also
slightly larger than the 40% of the population currently aged 1–30 that will
become the majority of the contributory population over the next three
decades.

The long (and increasing) life expectancies that Canadians enjoy and the relative size of the 31–60 age demographic wedge ensure that the number of people 65 years of age and older in Canada will double over the next thirty years. These factors on their own, however, do not determine the share of the population that will be in the 65-plus age group in the future. The size of the younger population relative to this rapidly growing older age group will be determined, in part, by the number of younger people already in Canada by both birth rates and net immigration. Given the number of people currently in the 30 and younger age group and the below-replacement-level birth rates that have prevailed in Canada for the past thirty years, without net immigration, the 65-plus population will increase from today's one in eight to one in four of Canada's population by 2030.

In terms of the relative size of the demographic wedge and the following age group, there is essentially a balance (43% to 40%). The issue is that today's population aged 31–60 accounts for 43% of the total population compared with a population aged 61–90 that accounts for only 15% of the total population. In thirty years, today's 1–30 age group (40% of the current population) will be paired with a 61–90 age group that accounts, without migration, for 27% of the 2030 population. This group will be asked to support almost twice the load for pay-as-you-go health care systems.

Theoretically, the growth in the 65-plus age group's share of the population can be reduced by an increase in the annual number of births; above-replacement-level birth rates contribute to a lowering of the average and median age of the population. Practically, however, the cradle does not offer much potential. First and fundamentally, an increase in birth rates to an above-replacement-level would counter a worldwide trend of dramatic declines in birth rates. Urban lifestyles and reproductive planning technology have led to birth rates as low as 1.1 children per woman in some countries. Second, the demographic wedge is rapidly aging out of the childbearing stage of the life cycle, and therefore is increasingly not susceptible to the incentives for having children. Third, a child born today will not be part of the health care contributory population for at least two decades; while in the long run increased birth rates will help achieve a better demographic balance, in the short term they do nothing to alter the ratio of the 65-plus population to the contributory population.

Net immigration, however, increases the size of the contributory population relative to the size of the 65-plus population. The age profiles of both immigrants to and emigrants from Canada are distinctly younger than those of Canada's resident population; the greater the margin between immigration and emigration, the slower the share of the 65-plus population grows. Achieving a 0.75% immigration rate and a 0.16% emigration rate will reduce the annual rate of increase of the contributory population's load from the average of 1.26% per year to 0.86% per year. If the federal target of 1.0% immigration is attained, the annual rate of increase of the contributory population's load will only be 0.74%.

Even with a 1.0% immigration rate, the annual increase in the real contribution required from each member of the 20–64 population resulting from demographic change alone will increase by almost twice the 0.43% per annum increase demographic change caused between 1975 and 1998. Without any change in spending patterns — without any change in today's health care system — we must anticipate an increase in the financial requirements needed to support provincial government spending. This increase will be between two and three times as great as the increases we have experienced over the past 25-odd years.

Demographics will not determine either the quality or the characteristics of Canadian health care in the future; these will be determined by how we respond to the pressures that demographic change — along with technological, social, economic, and environmental change — will bring.[20] What we cannot deny is that change will occur. An aging population does not necessarily bring increasing health care costs, but it does inevitably bring increasing health care costs if age-specific health care expenditures are not reduced. The logic is inescapable: with age-specific health care costs that increase steadily from the 5–9 age group, the faster the number of people in older age groups increases relative to the number of people in the younger age groups, and the greater the increase in real per capita health care spending unless age-specific spending is reduced.

Change the demographics, change the spending pattern, and a different scenario for the future emerges. It is a healthy sign that the health care debate is now shifting to focus on what changes are necessary and how they can be implemented. Examples of this focus are presented by an increasing number of authors, as evidenced by other contributions in this volume and in other reports and books. For example, the C.D. Howe Institute recently released a report on reforming health care financing in Canada; while the focus of the report is policy, the need for reform is based on a demographic projection similar to the one used here.[21]

Ready or not, change is coming to health care and to communities in

Canada. We can — and must — look to the experience and practice of other countries, to the proposals and concerns of health care providers and communities, and to the benefits and burdens that change will generate in order to prepare for change. But we must also look beyond the health care system itself to the economic and demographic change that can assist Canada in altering the health care system to ensure that it is one that will best serve us in the future.

NOTES

1. Canadian Institute for Health Information, "Data Tables Series E," *National Health Expenditure Trends, 1975–2000* (Ottawa: CIHI, 2000), 393–415.
2. Based on data from "Data Tables Series A," CIHI, *National Health Expenditure Trends,* 85.
3. Health Canada, *National Health Expenditures in Canada, 1975 to 1994* (Ottawa: Health Canada, 1996).
4. Based on analysis of data from Health Canada in David Baxter and Andrew Ramlo, *Healthy Choices: Demographics and Health Spending in Canada, 1980 to 2035* (Vancouver: The Urban Futures Institute, 1998).
5. Based on data from CIHI in *National Health Expenditure Trends.* These published data are for irregular age groups; estimates for the regular five-year age groups used here (which occur within the irregular age groups) were prepared by the author using unpublished data provided by the British Columbia Ministry of Health. Using the regular age groups provides a closer approximation of the timing of increases in provincial government spending.
6. Statistics Canada, "Immigration and Citizenship Table 1," *1996 Census National Series CD-ROM* (Ottawa: Statistics Canada, 1998).
7. Compiled from data published in Statistics Canada, *Vital Statistics: Births* (Ottawa: Statistics Canada, various years) and Statistics Canada, *Annual Demographic Statistics 1999 CD-ROM* (Ottawa: Statistics Canada, 2000).
8. Based on data from Statistics Canada, *Annual Demographic Statistics 1999.*
9. Based on data from CIHI, *National Health Expenditure Trends.*
10. Annual population data from Statistics Canada, *Annual Demographic Statistics 1999.*
11. Inflation data from Statistics Canada, "CANSIM Matrix 9940," *Consumer Price Index* (Ottawa: Statistics Canada, 2001).
12. Based on data from Statistics Canada, *Vital Statistics: Births* and Statistics Canada, *Annual Demographic Statistics 1999.*
13. Based on data from Statistics Canada, *Annual Demographic Statistics 1999.*
14. Based on data from Statistics Canada, *Annual Demographic Statistics 1999.*
15. Based on data from Statistics Canada, *Health Statistics at a Glance CD-ROM* (Ottawa: Statistics Canada, 1999).
16. All projections are from The Urban Futures Institute Population Projection Model. For discussion of methodology and background of this model, see David Baxter, Jim Smerdon, and Andrew Ramlo, *Forty Million: Canada's Population in the Next Four Decades* (Vancouver: The Urban Futures Institute, 1999). Specific values presented

here do not precisely match those in this earlier publication, as more recent data are used in this analysis.

17. Based on data from Statistics Canada, *Annual Demographic Statistics 1999*. For a discussion of the issues underlying immigration age profiles, see David Baxter, *Just Numbers: Demographic Change and Immigration in Canada's Future* (Vancouver: The Urban Futures Institute, 1998).

18. Based on data from Statistics Canada, *Annual Demographic Statistics 1999*.

19. Liberal Party of Canada Web site, *Multiculturalism — Our Direction*, www.liberal.ca/lpc/issuse.asp, 1 Feb. 2001.

20. For a discussion about the role that economic growth might play in supporting health care, see David Baxter, *A Prescription for Growth: The Demographic and Economic Context for Sustaining British Columbia's Health Care System* (Vancouver: The Urban Futures Institute, 2000).

21. William B.P. Robson, "Will the Baby Boomers Bust the Health Budget? Demographic Change and Health Care Financing Reform," *C.D. Howe Institute Commentary No. 148*, Feb. 2001. Released after this essay was completed, Robson's paper combines the same CIHI 1998 data used here with various population projections and economic trends to estimate the future demand for health care spending in relation to provincial revenues. He translates the increase in health's claims on budgets in the future into a present-value unfunded liability of between $500 and $800 billion. That amount rivals current federal and provincial debts in size, suggesting that current trends are not fiscally sustainable.

PART 4

HEATH CARE IN
AN INTERNATIONAL CONTEXT

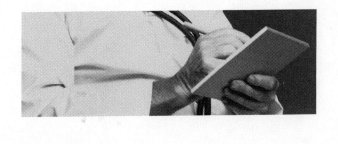

MYTHS ABOUT U.S. HEALTH CARE

David R. Henderson

Mention medicare and sooner rather than later, "it" comes up. "It," of course, is the *other* health care system. If Canadians are concerned about the state of their own system, they are equally concerned by what they perceive as inadequacies in the American one. But many of the beliefs that Canadians hold about U.S. health care — and, indeed, many of the beliefs that *Americans* hold about U.S. health care — are simply false. In this essay, Dr. David R. Henderson, an economist, describes American medicine.

He begins by considering a popularly stated fact: 43 million Americans are without health care. It's a myth, he argues, pointing out that these citizens are without insurance, not health care — an important distinction. Furthermore, he notes that the uninsured are typically without insurance for only a short time; only half of today's uninsured will be without insurance in five months.

If our understanding of the uninsured is misguided, so too is the Canadian belief that American health care represents a ruggedly free market. Henderson notes that "The U.S. medical system is one of the most regulated industries in the United States" and gives several examples of the government's heavy hand.

American employers provide their employees with health insurance partly because of government regulation. Henderson describes the skewed impact that nuances in the IRS code have on health delivery. Health insurance for the elderly and for the poor is entirely government-run. This is no small matter as these programs cover millions of citizens. And, as Henderson notes, the programs largely account for the explosion in health costs, even though they are subject to price controls implemented by the federal government.

Even the private insurance market is heavily regulated. Consider that state and federal regulations have effectively outlawed basic insurance. Mandated coverage includes liver transplants in Illinois, hairpieces in Minnesota, and sperm bank deposits in Massachusetts — these expensive mandates drive up the cost of insurance.

Government also plays a major role in determining physician supply, and in licensing doctors. Finally, Henderson observes that the Food and Drug Administration has a monopoly over the licensing of prescription drugs.

All of these observations lead Henderson to a simple point: "Will Rogers once said that it's not what we don't know that hurts us; rather, it's what we know that's not true. One reason Canadians have rejected free market solutions to their health care problems is that many of them think, as do many Americans, that the U.S. health care system is one of laissez-faire. It's not."

In 1971, I was twenty years old and living in Winnipeg. Dennis, a fellow Winnipegger who was itching to move to the United States, told me of a conversation he had had with his mother. His mother strenuously objected to his moving south, but he countered all her objections. Finally, in frustration, she said (obviously thinking that she had landed the knockout punch), "They don't have medicare down there. What will you do if you get sick?" Good question, I thought, not having considered the issue and not having a ready answer myself. But Dennis's immediate reply was, "I'll buy health insurance." I had quite literally never thought of that. Little was I to know that only about a year later I would be moving to the U.S. to go to graduate school, never to return to Canada for more than a few weeks at a time. Just as my friend Dennis had planned, I did get low-cost major medical insurance shortly after arriving in Los Angeles.

I'm reminded of this story when I think about the misunderstandings I regularly hear from Canadians about medical care and health insurance in the United States. Canadians believe many things about health care in the United States that are not true. This isn't surprising. Some of the main misconceptions that Canadians have about U.S. health care are ones they get from watching American television and reading American magazines and newspapers. In other words, some of the myths that Canadians believe about health care in the United States are also myths that Americans believe about their own health care system. How could it be that so many Americans are misinformed about their own system? Simple. If misconceptions are reported enough times, people start to believe them, even if those beliefs are belied by their personal experience.

The Myth That 43 Million Americans Are without Health Care

One of the main misconceptions is that about 43 million people in the United States, out of a population of about 280 million, go without health care. Turn on any talk show on American television in which people are discussing U.S. health care, and the odds are high that someone on the show will make such a statement. Sometimes the people who make the statement know better; sometimes they don't. But the truth is that very few people in the United States, if any, go without the health care they truly need. So where does the 43 million number come from? It's the number of people in the United States who, at any given time, are without *health insurance.*

But lacking health insurance and lacking health care are two very different things. Even if you lack health insurance, you have two other options. One is charity care, which doctors and hospitals in the United States have traditionally provided. The other is to pay for it yourself. The fact that you lack health insurance is not in itself evidence that you can't pay for health care. Most people who lack health insurance can afford to pay for basic health care and even those uninsured people who run up bills in the thousands of dollars due to a medical emergency can often arrange generous terms — including zero interest rates — for paying off those bills over years.

Moreover, since the 1980s, federal law has prohibited hospitals in the United States from turning away people who are having heart attacks or other life-threatening medical emergencies. Although this law may sound completely reasonable to many, there are two things to note about it. First, even before the law existed, very few people in dire straits were ever turned away from hospitals simply because they lacked health insurance. Second, the law has arguably reduced access to health care in areas where there is expected to be a large proportion of nonpayers. It has done so in two ways. First, the law caused some hospitals in inner cities to close down. Second, the law caused some hospitals to hide their trauma care entrances in order to discourage nonpaying customers. Both of these consequences were unintended, but were also entirely predictable to anyone who thought through the incentives the law created.

Many people believe that the 43 million uninsured people in the United States are the same people year-in, year-out. That belief is false. Imagine that Eastman Kodak invented a camera that could take a collective picture of those 43 million people and still show the detail of each person's face.

Let's say the camera takes a picture of those people and then takes a picture of the 43 million people who are without health insurance five months later. Question: What percentage of the people in the first photo are also in the second photo? Answer: About 50 percent. In other words, fully half of the people who lack health insurance at a given time have health insurance just five months later. Why do they go without health insurance for such a short time? Because most jobs in the United States carry health insurance for employees who want it, and many of the noninsured are people who are out of work. Because unemployment is short-term for most people who are unemployed in a given year — the median duration of unemployment in 1998, for example, was seven weeks[1] — going without health insurance is also a short-term situation. As for the 43 million uninsured, only 15 percent are still without health insurance two years later.[2] In other words, of the 280 million people in the United States, only 6.5 million of them — or under 2.5 percent of the population — lack health insurance for two years or more. If a similar percentage of the Canadian population lacked health insurance for two years or more, under 800,000 Canadian residents would lack health insurance for that time period.

The Myth That There is No Regulation of U.S. Health Care

The main other myth that Canadians hold about U.S. health care is that the U.S. has a free market system. This is untrue. The U.S. medical system is one of the most regulated industries in the United States. In fact, most of the problems that people point to in the U.S. medical system are caused by regulation; the parts of the system that work best are the least regulated. How is U.S. medicine regulated? With apologies to Elizabeth Barrett Browning, let me count the ways.

1. Health insurance is provided by employers partly because of government regulation.

The main way people get health insurance in United States is through an employer. This in itself is a historical accident, which is the product of two government acts: wage controls and income tax. During World War II, the federal government had imposed general wage controls on the economy. Thus, an employer who wanted to pay employees more than the controls allowed had to get the government's permission. In a dynamic economy, especially one in which the government is financing wartime spending by printing money, employers often do want to raise wages in order to keep more productive employees. Consequently, employers needed some legal way to pay employees more. The wage controls prevented employers from raising wages, but did not restrict them from increasing benefits. One obvious benefit employers could provide was health insurance, and that's what many of them began to do.

There was one other advantage to giving employees health insurance. Although the payments were deductible as expenses from the employer's taxable income, they did not count as taxable income to employees. So even after the wage controls of World War II ended, employers and employees found it mutually beneficial to keep health insurance as part of employee compensation. The Internal Revenue Service caught on and tried to tax the benefits as if they were taxable income. But, responding to employers' and employees' protests, Congress passed a law enshrining the tax-free status of health insurance.[3]

The tax avoidance benefit of health insurance is more pronounced at higher marginal tax rates. If the marginal tax rate is only 20 percent, then an employer and employee can avoid 20¢ in taxes by shifting $1 from pay into tax-free health insurance. But if the marginal tax rate is 40 percent, shifting that same $1 helps avoid 40¢ in taxes. Throughout the 1950s, 1960s, and 1970s (with one major interruption for the Johnson-Kennedy tax cut of 1964), marginal tax rates rose, making it increasingly attractive for employers to shift compensation from taxable money payments to nontaxable health insurance.

The main economist who drove home the crucial role of marginal tax rates in encouraging generous employer-provided health insurance was Harvard economist Martin Feldstein. He was chairman of President Reagan's Council of Economic Advisers when I was the Council's senior economist for health care policy. Feldstein gave examples like the following (updated with 2000 data): Consider an employer and an employee trying to decide on an extra dollar in taxable wages or an extra dollar of health insurance. The employee is earning, say, $40,000. If this employee has a spouse who earns $25,000, the family is likely to be in the 28 percent federal tax bracket. The social security tax rate (for employer and employee combined) is 12.4 percent. The Medicare tax rate (employer plus employee) is 2.9 percent. The employee's family is likely to be in at least a 5 percent marginal state income tax bracket. The marginal tax rate of this employee,

who is by no means unusual, is 28% + 12.4% + 2.9% + 3.6%,[4] for a whop-
ping total of 46.9%. Thus, almost half of an additional dollar of cash
compensation goes to various governments and it is this half that can be
avoided by taking additional compensation in health insurance rather than
in cash. As long as the employee values an extra $1 in health insurance at
more than about 53.1¢ (100 − 46.9) he or she is better off taking it in that
form. Health economists have pointed out that this is the main reason
employers have paid for insurance policies with low deductibles and low
copayment rates, the percentage of the bill paid by the patient. The employee
is better off to charge a $50 doctor's bill to the insurance company — even
if the company spends $20 to process it — and have the employer pay the
extra $70 in a higher premium to cover the bill and the processing cost.
The alternative — having the employer pay an extra $70 in cash — yields
the employee only about $42 and costs the employer $75.36 ($70 + $5.36,
the employer's portion of the social security and medicare tax on $70).

As a result, employees who spend on health care are mainly spending
other people's money. This is not to say that they are free riding. They are
not. Much of the money they spend on health insurance is their money;
they would have otherwise received it as higher wages and salaries. Nevertheless, once it is spent on insurance, it becomes other people's money.

Low deductibles have led people to think of health insurance not as
insurance at all, but as prepayment for unlimited medical care. Then, when
insurance companies try to tighten up and, for example, require their
beneficiaries to go to a cheaper doctor or to pay the difference if they want
to use an expensive doctor, the beneficiaries often howl. They are used to
having all their medical care paid for and don't like being asked to pay
more than a few hundred dollars out of their own pockets.

A typical copayment for a doctor's visit is 15 percent. Such low percentages give patients only a tiny incentive to shop for a lower-priced doctor. If,
for example, you can find a doctor who charges $50 for an office visit
instead of $70, you will not save $20 for yourself, but instead, will save $17
for the insurance company and only $3 for yourself. With such a small
savings, why bother shopping for the lower-priced doctor? In fact, the few
times I have ever asked the doctor's fee when calling to make an appointment, I was greeted by a tone of incredulity. The impression I got was that
almost no one ever asks. With very few customers searching for a lower
price, the result is that prices are higher than they otherwise would be.

Similarly, just as it is hard to get a price quote from a doctor, it is impossible to get a firm package price for surgery. Instead you get separate bills from the doctor, the other doctor, the hospital, and the anesthetist. And just try making sense of each item in a multicharge hospital bill. You may believe the reason behind the complexity is that medical care is in some way unique. But that idea doesn't hold up under close scrutiny. Consider cosmetic surgery, one of the few types of medical care not typically covered by health insurance. Health economist John Goodman writes:

> [E]ven though many parties are involved in supplying the service (physician, nurse, anesthetist, and the hospital), patients are quoted a single package price in advance. In other words, ordinary people, spending their own money, have been able to get advance price information that large employers, large insurance companies, and even federal and state governments generally have been unable to get for any other type of surgery.[5]

The key, therefore, is that people are spending their own money for plastic surgery and when they do, they exert a discipline on providers that does not exist otherwise.

2. Health insurance for the elderly and the poor is government-run.

The main other way people get health insurance is through Medicare, the government-run health insurance program for the elderly, and Medicaid, the government-run health insurance program for the poor and near-poor. Of course, by definition, these programs are the opposite of free market programs.

Under both Medicare and Medicaid, patients pay very little out-of-pocket. Under Medicaid, they usually pay nothing. Medicare beneficiaries pay a small percentage of doctors' fees; receive a large number of days in the hospital at no charge (after which they are responsible for all charges); and pay for their own prescription drugs. Because they pay so little for various costly medical services, they have little incentive to restrain their usage of medical care. The main disincentive is the value of their time. As a result, many beneficiaries of Medicare and of Medicaid use the medical system, not only for serious ailments, but also for minor ones.

Not surprisingly, therefore, these two programs are the main source of the explosion in U.S. health care costs. Both programs began in 1965. That's about when health care costs started rising dramatically. Between 1970 and 1999, government spending on Medicare and Medicaid grew from $12.3 billion to $403 billion. Adjusted for inflation, this is an increase of 663 percent.

During those same years, private spending grew from $46.7 billion to $662.1 billion. Adjusted for inflation, this is a 230 percent increase, or only about one-third of the growth in government spending.[6] When the Medicare law was passed in 1965, the House Ways and Means Committee forecasted that by 1990, annual spending for hospital care under Medicare would be $9.6 billion.[7] In fact, it turned out to be $67 billion.[8]

3. Under Medicare, the federal government imposes price controls on hospitals and doctors.

As one way to restrain spending in Medicare, the federal government imposed price controls on both hospitals and doctors. The price controls on hospitals came first. Beginning in 1983, the federal government started paying hospitals, not on the basis of cost reimbursement but, instead, on the basis of the diagnosis. The government came up with hundreds of possible diagnoses and set a price for each diagnosis-related group (DRG).

When the government sets a price that it, as the buyer, will pay, it is not necessarily deemed price control because setting a price doesn't preclude the patient from paying more. But what made it price control in this case is that the government forbade hospitals from "balance-billing," — that is, from charging an amount over and above the price it received from the federal government. DRG pricing was intended to cause, and may have caused, an increase in hospital efficiency. When hospitals were being reimbursed for their costs, they had little or no incentive to keep costs low. But when they were given a fixed price, they had a strong incentive to restrain costs. However, efficiency is not the only incentive effect of DRG pricing. There are two other potential effects. One is that the hospitals may discharge Medicare patients earlier than they would otherwise, and sometimes unsafely so. The second effect is that hospitals are thought to game the system by coming up with more than one diagnosis to get multiple payments, by choosing the diagnosis that maximizes the payment, and by discharging the patient and readmitting him or her later in order to receive payment for a new admission. A related effect is that the hospitals are thought to have unbundled their services as a way of keeping costs below the DRG price.

The government also restricts the fees that doctors may charge to Medicare patients and does not allow doctors to balance-bill. My conversations with doctors have led me to believe that they, as a result, limit the number of Medicare patients they will treat.

4. Private medical insurance is heavily regulated.

A bare-bones, high-deductible insurance policy that covers a large percentage of catastrophic expenses is fairly cheap. In 1991, for example, the *Wall Street Journal* reported on a Kansas plan with a $5,000 deductible that cost $900 a year.[9]

But state and federal regulation have made such bare-bones policies offered by employers illegal. Many states require employers who buy health insurance for their employees to also cover acupuncture, AIDS, alcoholism, drug abuse, and in vitro fertilization. Mandated coverages include heart transplants in Georgia, liver transplants in Illinois, hairpieces [!] in Minnesota, marriage counselling in California, and sperm bank deposits in Massachusetts.[10]

The federal government has three main mandates for employer-provided insurance. First, the federal Pregnancy Discrimination Act of 1978 requires employer-provided health insurance to cover pregnancy. MIT economist Jonathan Gruber has found that the 1978 law is mainly paid for out of the wages of female employees who are in their child-bearing years, which means that women who don't have children are implicitly subsidizing those who do.[11] Second, in the 1990s, the federal government began to dictate that employer-provided health insurance cover a minimum of forty-eight hours of hospital care for women giving vaginal birth. Third, it also began to require more expensive mental health coverage. As a result, an employee who doesn't want such coverage and an employer who doesn't want to provide it are out of luck. Instead of being able to offer a bare-bones health insurance policy at a modest cost and, therefore, at a modest reduction in wages, employers must offer an expensive program with an accompanying large cut in wages. (Interestingly, the people lobbying for these regulations are not groups of employees who want more coverage, but various associations of health care providers — chiropractors, mental health professionals, etc. — who want to create an artificial demand for their services.)

The way out is not to offer health insurance benefits at all; many employers of low-wage earners, for whom an expensive health insurance policy would mean a large percentage cut in wages, have opted not to insure their employees.

Another barrier to low-cost insurance in some states is the regulation of insurance policies sold to individuals. Two specific regulations in particular cause problems and, when combined, often cause the price of insurance for families to be more than $10,000 a year. The regulations I refer to are community rating and guaranteed issue.

Under *community rating*, insurers are not allowed to vary their premiums according to gender, age, occupation, or any of the other characteristics that affect the probability that their customers will use medical care once insured. This regulation is like requiring that auto insurance companies charge twenty-one-year-old males the same premiums as forty-year-old males. Because the rates must cover all the insurers' costs, including the expected payout, the rates are a bad deal for the healthy and a good deal for the less healthy. As a result, healthy people are less likely to buy insurance and less healthy people are more likely to buy insurance. The mix of the insured thus shifts toward the unhealthy, driving up premiums further, making it even less attractive for the healthy to buy insurance. The economic term for this effect is "adverse selection," so called because the mix of the insured is adverse to the insurance company. Interestingly, economists have written a great deal about how adverse selection is caused by asymmetric information — that is, by the potential buyer knowing more about his health status than the seller does. But this adverse selection is caused by government policy. With virtual unanimity, these economists believe that adverse selection due to asymmetric information is bad, which means they favour insurers charging different prices for different risks. Yet economists have been less outspoken in their criticism of community rating.

The other regulation, *guaranteed issue*, requires the insurance company to insure all comers. On its own, this regulation does little harm as long as an insurance company is free to price the insurance according to the risk. So, for example, someone with AIDS who wants insurance will be able to get it, but only by paying an extremely high premium. The moral of the story for the insurance buyer is that you shouldn't let guaranteed issue lull you into waiting until you're sick before you buy insurance.

But guaranteed issue combined with community rating has devastating consequences. If insurers must provide coverage to all comers and cannot price accordingly, then people will tend to wait until they get sick before they buy coverage. Knowing this, insurance companies raise their rates, making it even less attractive for the healthy to buy insurance. This disincentive causes many of them to drop out, which pushes rates even higher.

The whole set-up reminds me of an episode from the television show, *Cheers.* Bartender Woody develops a system for betting on football games;

he tests his system over a few weeks and finds that it works. He asks Sam for the name of a bookie so that he can bet $1,000. Not wanting Woody to lose his money, Sam tells him that he'll place the bet, but puts the money in his safe instead. Of course, Woody's predictions turn out to be right and he approaches Sam for his $30,000 winnings. Sam frantically schemes with Diane to come up with some way of getting the money.

Diane says, "Wait. I've got it."

"What?" asks Sam with panicked hope.

"Just go to the bookie," says Diane, "and explain the situation. I'm sure he'll understand."

Diane's solution is like waiting until you're sick to buy insurance. The difference is that *Cheers* is a comedy show and destructive insurance regulations affect real people. In the seven states where the community rating and guaranteed issue regulations are combined — New Jersey, New York, Washington, Kentucky, Vermont, Maine, and New Hampshire — there have been huge increases in premiums, hundreds of thousands of individuals have dropped their coverage, and the insurance market has dried up. In New York, for example, insurance premiums increased by 50 percent or more.[12] The fact that many firms left the insurance market in New York and every other state where these "reforms" were tried means that these premium increases were not a big benefit to the insurance companies but, rather, the result of the higher riskiness of the patient pool. One insurance agent I spoke to speculated that politicians and other government officials who support these regulations understand these effects and want them, so that they can cause more people to go without insurance and thus create a demand for government-provided insurance. I think his speculation is warranted.

5. Governments in the United States limit the number of doctors.

In late 1972, a few months after I arrived in Los Angeles and had bought my health insurance policy, I came down with a bad sore throat that would not go away. My doctor recommended a tonsillectomy, which I proceeded to have. Because my sore throat was a preexisting condition under the insurance company's rules, I had to pay the hospital and doctor's bill myself. The total was about $1,000, a large amount in 1972 dollars, which I borrowed from my father. A few weeks later, I attended the American Economics Association meetings in Toronto, where I ran into two of my favourite economics professors from my previous year at the University of Western Ontario. When I vented about the high cost, one of my former professors grinned at the other, looked at me and said, "You're experiencing life under the free market system you've been advocating."

"No, I'm not," I responded. "The U.S. system is highly regulated. And the regulations that really cost me are the ones that limit entry into the medical profession."

For the last century, state licensing boards in the United States have set tight standards that have resulted in a limit on the number of doctors. As with any good or service, when the supply is kept low, prices rise. Indeed, Milton Friedman, in his Ph.D dissertation (later made into a book), was the first economist to establish empirically that doctors' high pay is due to the limit on supply.[13]

Few people deny that the tight restrictions on entry into the medical profession have made doctors' salaries and fees substantially higher than they would be otherwise. What concerns many people, though, is whether we can have quality control without such restrictions. And we can, with a system of certification. Pop quiz: What two letters on the electrical equipment I use make me feel confident that I won't electrocute myself? Answer: UL, short for Underwriters' Laboratory.

Underwriters' Laboratory is a completely private organization that, for a fee, tests and certifies the safety of various items. The fact that it charges a fee to the manufacturers whose products it certifies creates an inherent conflict of interest. But UL is aware of this fact and, to offset it, has representatives of insurance companies on its board. The insurance companies have a strong incentive to make sure that UL doesn't certify something that isn't safe because unsafe products cost insurance companies money. Similarly, with or without government certification, if we eliminate licensing barriers from the medical professions, we would start to see private agencies that would certify the qualifications of medical professionals.

In fact, there are groups already in existence that are ready to become private certifiers. They're called managed care organizations (MCOs). Most MCOs don't actively judge the quality of doctors; they don't have to because state government agencies perform that task. But with the government out of that business, MCOs would have an incentive to take its place. In fact, one of the oldest and most well-known MCOs, Kaiser Permanente, has been certifying doctors for years. Interestingly, Milton Friedman points out in his 1962 classic, *Capitalism and Freedom*, that with private certification, medical teams can form. These teams have the potential to be, in his words, "department stores of medicine."[14] Just as department stores implicitly — and usually explicitly — guarantee the quality of the goods they sell, so would "department stores of medicine." This evolution is happening even with government licensing, making government certification irrelevant. The problem is that government licensing also restricts people from practising and does so not in response to a market test, but due to the political power held by doctors.

The problems with government licensing will become more obvious over the next few years because state restrictions will slow down — and sometimes prevent — the medical progress that the Internet is creating. It is now possible for a patient in, say, Davenport, IA to be diagnosed by a doctor in, say, Baltimore, MD. However, state licensing agencies are getting in the way, insisting that a doctor who practises on the Web is really practising in the state where his or her patient resides and must therefore meet that state's licensing standards.[15] But a private certifier will likely operate nationwide rather than statewide and would therefore not get in the way of such progress.

6. The Food and Drug Administration has monopoly power over the licensing of prescription drugs.

The government prevents competition in the pharmaceutical industry in two ways, the first of which has mainly good effects and the second of which has mainly bad effects. The restriction with good effects is the patent system. The government grants patents to drug developers that give them a legal monopoly for seventeen years. Without the prospect of a patent as its reward, a firm would not have nearly enough incentive to spend the hundreds of millions of dollars needed to develop a single drug, which would undermine the innovation needed to produce the wonder drugs of today and tomorrow. The other way the government prevents competition and drives up the price of drugs is, however, unjustified and has caused the unnecessary early death of tens of thousands of people. Here I refer to regulation by the Food and Drug Administration (FDA).

Almost any American born before the middle of the twentieth century remembers the story of thalidomide, a drug administered in the late 1950s to help pregnant women with morning sickness. The drug had one horrible side effect: it caused some babies to be born with deformed limbs.

188 ◆ BETTER MEDICINE

Because of the thalidomide tragedy, the FDA was given new power (under the 1962 Kefauver amendments to the law) to regulate new drugs not just for safety — a power it had held since 1938 — but also for efficacy. Do you notice how strange this is? First, the thalidomide tragedy represents a partial failure of regulation: thalidomide was approved by the very agency that had the power to prevent unsafe drugs from being marketed. It's true that the FDA official in charge of the new drug application for thalidomide, Frances Kelsey, MD, was concerned about other possible effects of the drug, and her concern held up FDA approval for one year.[16] But the birth defects were discovered in Europe, not the U.S., so it was sheer luck — not careful regulation — that held the drug up here. Second, the thalidomide episode was used as an excuse for efficacy standards, even though the problem with thalidomide was safety, not efficacy.

Economists have found in countless studies that the efficacy regulations on drugs have delayed the introduction of new drugs by years and have added hundreds of millions of dollars to the cost of developing typical new drugs. Santa Clara University economics professor Daniel Klein surveyed all the economics studies that he could find on the effect of FDA regulation. He found that they were all critical of the extent of the FDA's absolute regulatory power over new drugs.[17] In a study of forty-six new drugs approved by the FDA in 1985 and 1986, for example, researchers at Tufts University's Center for Drug Development found that thirty-three were available, on average, 5.5 years later than in foreign markets.[18] Some medicines that are useful only for a few people, so-called "orphan" drugs, won't make enough money to compensate for the costs involved in meeting the FDA's testing requirements. Thus, we will forever be forbidden to use them, courtesy of the FDA.

These delays are killing people. In December 1988, for example, the FDA approved Misoprostol, a drug that prevents the gastric ulcers caused by aspirin and other nonsteroidal anti-inflammatory drugs. In some other countries, Misoprostol was available as early as 1985. Using the FDA's own estimates, Sam Kazman, an FDA expert at the Competitive Enterprise Institute, a public interest lobby in Washington, concluded that Misoprostol would have saved 8,000–15,000 lives a year.[19] Thus, the FDA's delay cost over 20,000 and as many as 50,000 innocent lives. And this is the cost of delay for only one out of hundreds of drugs. Economist Dan Klein estimates that FDA regulation kills about 50,000 people a year.[20]

And these regulations are not necessary. The FDA may have some expertise when it comes to drug safety and efficacy, but on the only issue that matters — your own tradeoffs among various risks — you are the expert, and the FDA's scientists are rank amateurs. One of my former undergraduate students, Charles Hooper, now a partner in the biotech consulting firm Objective Insights, writes:

> The choice a patient makes among therapies (with the help of his agent, the doctor) is based on many variables: efficacy, tolerability, side effects, riskiness, monetary cost, non-monetary cost (e.g., hassle), speed of action. These drug costs and benefits must be judged within the context of many personal values and tradeoffs: the fear of death, the fear of surgery, the fear of the hospital, potential pain, and the individual's health profile, financial status, value of time, value of health, and risk tolerance. For the FDA to decide what compounds pass this complex tradeoff is preposterous, given that the FDA can never frame the problem from the individual patient's perspective. One individual's best alternative could be another's worst. We have seen this with AIDS patients: "I don't care if I develop cancer and this costs me $20,000 a year because without it I'm dead in 6 months." If, instead of medical therapies, they were telling us what kind of washing machines to buy or where to go on vacation, we would consider it laughable. Centralized bureaucrats cannot make the proper decisions for individuals because they lack the requisite information.[21]

Consider the FDA's July 2000 ban on the drug Propulsid (a heartburn remedy) after the FDA linked it to dangerous irregular heartbeats in 340 people, of whom 80 died. Sounds reasonable to ban the drug, right? It turns out, though, that for some people with cerebral palsy, Propulsid was a godsend. One patient, twenty-two-year-old Rob O'Neill, began to moan in pain when digesting his food because the government forbade him from taking Propulsid, the only drug that had worked to help him digest.[22] It's true that the FDA will still allow the drug to be sold to some patients, but the agency insists that they meet strict criteria and be placed in special scientific studies. Of course, these restrictions raise the cost to the patients and the drug companies, making it less worthwhile to provide the drug at all, and certainly less worthwhile to find new users for it. Peanuts can kill people; these people typically know who they are and can avoid peanuts. But we don't ban peanuts just because they can kill some people. Interestingly, if peanuts were a drug, the FDA would probably ban them.

The solution, both for safety and for lower-cost, readily available drugs, is to strip the FDA of its absolute regulatory power over drugs and let any patient use any drug that a doctor is willing to prescribe. The FDA would then be a certifier of drugs, but not a regulator. Any drug not certified by the FDA would have to carry a warning label, similar to the one that appears on a cigarette package, saying, "WARNING: This drug has not been certified by the FDA."

When you read economics journals or textbooks or hear economists talk, you'll sometimes encounter the term "Pareto-optimal." This term describes a change, usually in government policy, that makes some people better off and no one worse off. In the real world, you'll find few such changes. The one I just proposed comes close. Divide drug buyers into two groups: those who want the options the FDA denies them, and those who want only the options the FDA certifies. By making the FDA a certifier instead of a regulator, those in the first group would have new choices and would thus be better off. Those in the second group would turn down those new choices and would thus be unaffected. Of course, the one group that *would* be hurt by the change is made up of the FDA employees who would lose much of their power over the drug companies. You have to attend just one FDA hearing (I testified at one in 1995) to know that many of these employees treasure their power to make drug companies do their bidding.

Moreover, I confidently predict that, if the FDA were made just a certifier rather than a regulator, virtually all patients and doctors would begin to trust alternate sources of information. What sources? There are many. In Europe, the European Agency for the Evaluation of Medicinal Products (EMEA) competes with national agencies of various European countries, so that a drug company in a given country can decide whether to go through that country's own agency or the EMEA. Currently in the United States, doctors often rely on private certifiers, such as the American Hospital Formulary Service.

Indeed, the reason I'm so confident that virtually every doctor would prescribe drugs not certified by the FDA is that virtually every doctor does so today. When the FDA allows a drug to be sold, it certifies the drug for specific uses. But no law prevents doctors from prescribing the drug for other uses not listed on the label. And doctors often find such "off-label" uses. Sometimes these off-label uses are obvious, and doctors discover them on their own and publicize their findings in medical journals. If, for example, a drug is certified for short-term treatment of a disease, it's not a big stretch to try it for long-term treatment. Other times, the drug company sponsors scientific studies to find new uses and then publicizes the results. A study begun in 1989, for example, found that Eli Lilly's antidepression drug, Prozac, was effective in treating premenstrual syndrome. According to Donald R. Bennett, MD, Ph.D, director of the American Medical Association's Division of Drugs and Toxicology at the time, between 40 and 50 percent of all drugs are prescribed for off-label use. Between 60 and 70 percent of drugs used to treat cancer and 90 percent of drugs used in pediatrics are prescribed for off-label use.[23]

So what? The fact that virtually all doctors prescribe drugs for off-label use means, as health economist Alex Tabarrok has pointed out, that we already know that private certification works.[24]

The Myth That Managed Care Doesn't Work

In the last ten years, so-called managed care organizations have hugely expanded their market in U.S. private health care. In 1990, according to Northwestern University health economist David Dranove, 33.6 million Americans were enrolled in Health Maintenance Organizations (HMOs), the earliest form of MCOs, and today over 80 percent of working Americans are enrolled in some kind of managed care plan. Not everyone is happy with managed care. Yet, when you ask people why they don't like it, they don't usually give clear answers. They've read the horror stories about the substitution of a generic drug for a brand name drug saving a few dollars and costing a life. And they can quote a scene out of the movie *As Good As It Gets* in which actress Helen Hunt's onscreen sickly son gets truly lousy health care from an MCO. But they can't typically quote any careful studies showing that managed care leads to lower quality, and they haven't had particularly bad experiences themselves.

In his recent book, *The Economic Evolution of American Health Care: From Marcus Welby to Managed Care*, Dranove makes the case, datum by datum, that managed care organizations have "managed" to cut costs without noticeably hurting the quality of health care.[25] While MCOs were gaining share in the 1990s, notes Dranove, private sector health care spending rose by only 5 percent a year. That may not sound like much of an accomplishment. But Dranove points out that at the start of the 1990s, before MCOs took over, health care spending was rising by more than 10 percent a year and the Congressional Budget Office predicted in 1993 that by 2000, health care spending would be 18.9 percent of GDP. Instead, it has remained below 14 percent, where it was seven years ago. Even more striking is that the cost savings have occurred almost entirely in the private sector, which is where managed care has taken over. Private sector health care spending is now $300 billion less annually than it was projected to be. This amounts to a cool $2,000 a year in savings per privately insured patient. Medicare spending, by contrast, grew at twice the rate of private spending during the 1990s.

How did managed care achieve such savings? Essentially by setting up incentives for certain players in the health care system to say "no" to more health care spending. Previously, no one had that role. Before MCOs, insured patients knew that they would pay little or nothing out-of-pocket when they saw a doctor, got a test, or were admitted to a hospital. Doctors often had a financial incentive to order more tests and to practise what Dranove and other health care economists call flat-of-the-curve medicine (spending large amounts of money for very small increments of health). Insurance companies passively paid the bills. But as technology developed and spending grew, insurance companies raised premiums, upsetting employers and, occasionally, employees who saw their money wages rise more slowly. Along came MCOs to place limits on tests and specialist visits and to drive down prices paid to doctors, drug companies, and hospitals. For reasons noted earlier, patients had very little reason to be sensitive to doctors' fees, but insurance companies did. And they have bargained many of those fees down. In some managed care settings, a primary care doctor was paid a fixed fee per patient per year. If a patient did not make a visit in a particular year, the doctor kept the entire fee; if the doctor sent a patient to a specialist, the specialist's fee was subtracted from the primary care doctor's revenues. Thus, for the first time, primary care doctors had a strong incentive to be frugal with medical services.

You might think that the new incentive would cause doctors to make serious cuts in quality. But most surveys, notes Dranove, find that HMO enrollees and enrollees in traditional "indemnity insurance" are about equally satisfied with the quality of their health care. Of course, survey data are notoriously unreliable. But other analysts who have compared quality between MCOs and traditional fee-for-service find that in some cases, HMOs are better when it comes to things like ordering mammography and colon cancer screening more frequently.

Why, if managed care is working reasonably well, is there such animus against it? Dranove points out that much of the opposition comes from providers, especially doctors, who are losing some autonomy and some income due to managed care. Interestingly, support for his thesis comes from California voters. In the mid-1990s, they got to vote on two laws that would have regulated MCOs. Voters rejected them by 58% vs. 42% and 61% vs. 39%. That's why the only headway being made to regulate HMOs is being made in legislatures, where lobbies of nurses and doctors are spearheading the regulatory push. Another source of the opposition to managed care, speculates Dranove, is that it *is* working well and is therefore making it harder for advocates of socialized medicine to push their case.

Fortunately, there is a safety valve with managed care. If you don't like the fact that managed care won't pay for a test that you or your doctor thinks is a good idea, you are free to get the test and pay for it yourself. This is a freedom that people in countries with socialized medicine, including Canada, often don't have.

Conclusion

Will Rogers once said that it's not what we don't know that hurts us; rather, it's what we know that's not true. One reason Canadians have rejected free market solutions to their health care problems is that many of them think, as do many Americans, that the U.S. health care system is one of laissez-faire. It's not. And most of the problems in U.S. health care that upset people are caused by, or are exacerbated by, government regulation. Indeed, the parts of the U.S. health care system that work best are those that are least regulated.

So what should Canadians do to get out of the socialized medical mess without falling into the subsidized, regulated U.S. mess? Two reforms, taken together, would go a long way to give Canadians the power to make their own medical choices, a power they have not had in over thirty years.

The first reform involves stopping the government from preventing the purchase of medical care. Anyone who wants medical care and anyone who wants to sell it should be free to do so. That way, if a woman wants to avoid the joys of natural childbirth and is willing to pay an anesthetist for an epidural, she would be free to do so and the anesthetist would be free to offer the service at a market rate. Or, if someone wants a CT scan and doesn't want to wait months for the socialized medical sector to provide it, he would be free to use his own money to pay for the test.

The second reform — introducing medical savings accounts (MSAs) — would make it easier for people to purchase health care and wean themselves off medicare. The idea here is that people and/or their employers would be free to put aside a certain amount of before-tax funds every year to be spent on health insurance premiums, deductibles, copayments, and noncovered services. A reasonable amount would be $4,000 to $5,000 annually. To give people an incentive not to spend the money without good reason, the government could let them accumulate unspent sums and invest them in interest-bearing assets. They could then draw on these funds when they retire. It's the same principle as the one behind U.S. Individual Retirement Accounts (IRAs) and Canadian Registered Retirement Savings Plans (RRSPs).

Consider an employee with MSA money who is trying to choose between two insurance policies. The first is a catastrophic policy with an annual deductible of, say, $1,500 a year and an annual premium of, say, $2,000 a year. The second is a policy with an annual deductible of $300 a year and a premium of $2,800 a year. The employee knows that the money being spent on insurance is his or her own. That employee would therefore be careful when choosing between the policies. Many employees would choose the catastrophic policy and as a result, they would be spending their own money (at least for the first $1,500) when purchasing health care. This personal expenditure would encourage cost-consciousness and, in turn, bring a consumer-driven discipline to the medical marketplace that does not presently exist.

NOTES

1. This datum is from Hoyt Bleakley, Ann Ferris, and Jeffrey Fuhrer, "In a Booming Economy, Unemployment has Remained Surprisingly High," Federal Reserve Bank of Boston Regional Review, No. 4, 1999, www.bos.frb.org/economic/nerr/rr1999/q4/issu99_4.htm.
2. These data are from Katherine Swartz and Timothy D. McBride, "Spells Without Health Insurance: Distribution and Their Link to Point-in-Time Estimates of the Uninsured," Inquiry 27 (Fall, 1990): 281–88.
3. See Milton Friedman, "The Folly of Buying Health Care at the Company Store," Wall Street Journal, 3 Feb. 1993.
4. If the family itemizes its deductions on its federal tax form, it can deduct its state income taxes. Therefore, the family's 5% tax rate, after taking account of deductibility, is really 3.6% [(1 − .28) * 5%].
5. See John C. Goodman, "Health Insurance," in David R. Henderson, ed., The Fortune Encyclopedia of Economics (New York: Warner Books, 1993), 684–89.
6. Data on rates of expenditure growth from Suzanne W. Letsch, Helen C. Lazenby, Katharine R. Levit, and Cathy A. Cowan, "National Health Expenditures, 1991," Health Care Financing Review, 14 (Winter 1992): 18. Updated data from www.hcfa.gov/stats. Adjustments for inflation made using the Consumer Price Index.

7. House Committee on Ways and Means, Public Law 89–97, 98th Congress, 1st Session (30 July 1965), 33, cited in Peter J. Ferrara, "The Clinton/Gephardt Bill," *Policy Backgrounder No. 133* (Dallas: National Center for Policy Analysis, 1994), 14.

8. *1994 Annual Report of the Board of Trustees of the Federal Hospital Insurance Trust Funds*, Washington, DC, 11 Apr. 1994, in Ferrara, "The Clinton/Gephardt Bill."

9. Hilary Stout, "Moves to Ease Health-Insurance Rules Criticized," *Wall Street Journal*, 4 June 1991.

10. Facts taken from John C. Goodman and Gerald L. Musgrave, *Patient Power: Solving America's Health Care Crisis* (Washington: Cato Institute, 1992), 324–25.

11. Jonathan Gruber, "The Efficiency of a Group-Specific Mandated Benefit: Evidence from Health Insurance Benefits for Maternity," working paper no. 4157, National Bureau of Economic Research, Sept. 1992.

12. Bureau of National Affairs, "New York State to Use Insurance Pool Funds to Avert Major Health Premium Increases," *Health Care Policy* 6 (27 Apr. 1998).

13. Milton Friedman and Simon Kuznets, *Income from Independent Professional Practice* (New York: National Bureau of Economic Research, 1945).

14. Milton Friedman, *Capitalism and Freedom* (Chicago: University of Chicago Press, 1962), 159.

15. See Bill Richards, "Hold the Phone: Doctors Can Diagnose Illnesses Long Distance, To the Dismay of Some," *Wall Street Journal*, 17 Jan. 1996, A1.

16. For the full story, see Steven B. Harris, MD, "The Right Lesson to Learn from Thalidomide," at www.aces.uiuc.edu:8001/Liberty/Tales/Thalidomide.html.

17. Daniel Klein, "Economists Against the FDA," *Ideas on Liberty*, Sept. 2000, 18–21.

18. See K.I. Kaitin, B.W. Richard, and Louis Lasagna, "Trends in Drug Development: The 1985–86 New Drug Approvals," *Journal of Clinical Pharmacology* 27 (Aug. 1987): 542–48.

19. Sam Kazman, "Deadly Overcaution: FDA's Drug Approval Process," *Journal of Regulation and Social Costs* 1 (Aug. 1990): 42–3.

20. Klein, "Economists Against the FDA."

21. Charles Hooper, letter to author, 18 Sept. 1995.

22. "Drug Ban Brings Misery to Patient," Associated Press, 11 Nov. 2000.

23. The data and source are cited in Andrew A. Skolnick, "Pro-Free Enterprise Group Challenges FDA's Authority to Regulate Drug Companies' Speech," *Journal of the American Medical Association* (2 Feb. 1994).

24. Alex Tabarrok, "Assessing the FDA via the Anomaly of Off-Label Drug Prescribing," *The Independent Review*, Summer 2000, 25–53.

25. See David Dranove, *The Economic Evolution of Health American Health Care: From Marcus Welby to Managed Care* (Princeton: Princeton University Press, 2000).

ACCESSIBLE, HIGH-QUALITY, AND COST-EFFECTIVE HEALTH CARE: A PUBLIC OR PRIVATE MATTER?

Cynthia Ramsay

Canadians hear relatively little about how other countries organize their health care systems. More troubling still, international comparisons are typically done through the myopic prism of nationalism ("we have the best health care system in the world") or with simplistic comparisons (infant mortality rates, for example). In this essay, health economist Cynthia Ramsay looks at the health care systems abroad and then describes them in a major comparative study.

Ramsay focuses on eight countries, "chosen for study because they represent a spectrum of public and private sector delivery and financing of health care." They include Canada, the United States, Germany, Switzerland, the United Kingdom, Australia, Singapore, and South Africa.

Ramsay begins by describing the different organizational structures. Several countries have systems built on the British National Health Service (NHS) model, such as Canada, Australia, and South Africa. Though they share a common history, these three health care systems have evolved differently. In Australia, for example, physicians can extra-bill and patients can opt out of the public system. In Canada, extra-billing and private insurance aren't allowed.

Health care in other countries (particularly in Germany and Switzerland) is based on the idea of a social insurance. The private sector plays a large role in medical care in the United States and Singapore, but the system in both countries is heavily influenced by government regulation and legislation.

International comparisons are often performed casually, but there is actually a limited body of meaningful work. Ramsay describes the much publicized World Health Organization (WHO) study that ranked Canada 30th of 191 countries in terms of overall health system performance. She then explains her own study, which took more than a year to complete. Based on over 100 separate variables grouped into 17 categories including health coverage, preventable illness, and equality, Ramsay compares eight nations.

Ramsay describes her findings, focusing on three supercategories for health care: quality, access, and cost. While Canada does well on the second, other countries outperform us in the other two areas. Overall, Canada ranks midpack. Depending on preference for public funding or private financing, the United Kingdom or Singapore ranks first.

Ramsay concludes: "Contrary to the common belief in Canada, the health index scores demonstrate that either a publicly or privately funded health care system can deliver timely, quality medical care to all citizens. . . . As well, Canada is not the only country in the world that values universality. In terms of access to care, all eight countries have measures that attempt to ensure that their citizens receive health care when they need it, regardless of their ability to pay. Conversely, no system has successfully eliminated inequalities in health status across socioeconomic or racial groups."

1. Introduction

Canada has had some form of publicly funded health care for more than three decades — longer if we include hospital insurance. The general feeling has been that a publicly funded system is necessary to ensure that all Canadians receive quality health care whenever they need it.

The 2001 federal Throne Speech states that "medicare, which ensures access to needed services regardless of income or place of residence, is vital to our quality of life."[1] Federal Health Minister Allan Rock asserts that the "vast majority of Canadians cherish our single-payer, publicly administered health care system. . . ."[2] The 1999–2000 annual report of the Canada Health Act claims that medicare has "iconic status for Canadians."[3]

Yet several factors have been putting pressure on the system for years: the need for government fiscal responsibility, an aging population, the cost of new medical technologies, increasing demand for health care in general, and so on. Now the norm is increased waiting times for surgical treatment, overcrowded emergency rooms, limits on the amount of specialized care available, nursing shortages, and physician strikes.

In light of these problems, Canadians are questioning whether medicare is providing access to needed services. In 1999, the Commonwealth Fund surveyed public satisfaction with health care systems in Canada, the United Kingdom, the United States, Australia, and New Zealand. The study found that of these five countries, Canada had the largest loss of public confidence in their health system from 1988 to 1998.[4] A January 2000 Reuters news service press story asked, "What on earth has happened to Canada's health service, which many Canadians once assumed was the envy of the world?"[5]

In response to growing national discontent, various levels of government in Canada have conducted numerous royal commissions, forums, and studies on health care. The result has been a lot of talk about reform, but very few major reforms have actually been implemented.

One of the barriers to change seems to be the prevalent attitude that anyone who wishes to alter the current system significantly is one of medicare's "enemies." These "enemies" are depicted as "powerful economic interests" who want Canada to "drift down the road taken by the United States . . . a maelstrom of increasing inefficiency and inequity, and ever-increasing cost. . . ."[6]

Setting aside the question of whether such characterizations are valid, there is the larger issue of why any reform proposals that include an increased role for the private sector are perceived as an effort to "Americanize" the Canadian health care system. Every industrialized country except Canada permits the purchase or sale of private insurance for medical services covered by government insurance. As well, most countries in the world are committed to the principle of accessible, timely, quality medical care being provided to *all* residents, regardless of their ability to pay for needed care. Canada does not have a monopoly on the concept of universality.

If Canadians are to successfully improve their system, they must start by abandoning these two misconceptions: that the United States is the only other health system model and that Canada's principles regarding health care are unique.

To aid in this process, I conducted a study for the Calgary-based Marigold Foundation entitled "Beyond the Public-Private Debate: An Examination of Quality, Access and Cost in the Health Care Systems of Eight Countries." For more than a year, from November 1999 to December 2000, I gathered data on the delivery and financing of health care in Canada, the United States, Germany, Switzerland, the United Kingdom, Australia, Singapore, and South Africa. These data, based on more than 100 variables and grouped into 17 broad categories, were used to compare the health care systems of the countries. The countries were then ranked, using a focus of quality, access, and cost of health care (see section 4 of this essay for a more detailed presentation of the study). Throughout the research process, I consulted many experts in economics and health care.

Although any results should be interpreted as general findings rather than specific conclusions, it is still useful to make international comparisons and several organizations have done so despite the shortcomings of the data. (For example, the UN Human Development Index ranks countries according to several variables, such as their wealth and social equality; yet, for many countries, little or no data are available for several of the variables.)

2. Comparing Health Systems

The eight countries studied were chosen because they represent a spectrum of public and private sector delivery and financing of health care. Of these countries, private funding plays the largest role in Singapore, yet that country's government is very active in directing the health care system. The private sector provides the majority of health care funding in the United States and South Africa, while the United Kingdom, Canada, Australia, Germany, and Switzerland rely more on public sector funding.

Many of these countries share a common origin and, hence, some common traits — the United Kingdom's National Health Service (NHS) influenced the formation of the Canadian, Australian, and South African health care systems. As well, seven of the eight countries are developed, wealthy nations, with relatively similar public health — access to clean water, proper sanitation systems, and absence of war and famine. In addition to its NHS-related history, South Africa is included in the study in order to capture the range of socioeconomic conditions within which health care systems must operate.

This section provides an overview of the different health care systems.

Canada

Canada has a predominant publicly financed, privately delivered health care system. There are certain services — those deemed medically necessary — that provincial governments are responsible for financing and for which every Canadian resident is provided insurance by the public sector. As well, most hospitals in Canada are government-financed. Private insurance for publicly funded health services is not permitted in Canada, but people are allowed to pay for those services not insured by the public sector.

Canada's current health system has its origins in the 1948 Hospital Construction Grants Program, in which the federal government made grants available to the provinces for planning and hospital construction. Under this legislation, the federal government completely funded the building of hospitals virtually anywhere in the country. Soon thereafter, provinces were insuring their citizens for hospital-based services.

In 1966, medical services provided by a physician became insured by a federal-provincial cost-sharing program as laid out in the Medical Care Act (implemented in 1968). To qualify for federal funding, a province's program had to be *universal* (cover all residents of a province), *portable* (cover residents of one province requiring medical services in another province), *comprehensive* (cover all medically necessary services), and *publicly administered* (a not-for-profit program). The Canada Health Act (1984) added another requirement to the Medical Care Act: *accessibility*.

The federal government tries to achieve accessibility by reducing its payments to the provinces, on a dollar-for-dollar basis, by the amount of user fees charged by hospitals and extra-billing by physicians. It is not possible for the federal government to directly prohibit these types of charges, as health care is officially a provincial responsibility.

The public sector — federal, provincial, and municipal governments and the Workers' Compensation Boards — accounted for 69.4 percent of total health care spending in 1997; the private sector — households and businesses — accounted for the other 30.6 percent.[7] Governments pay mainly for medically necessary services (that is, acute care, physicians' fees, and a portion of pharmaceutical, dental, and eye care charges), however, as there is no definition as to what constitutes "medically necessary," each province has its own health insurance plan and that covers different services to different extents. While some doctors are paid by salary, most doctors in Canada are independent practitioners who provide services to their patients and then are paid on a fee-for-service basis by the government; most nurses are paid on a salaried basis.

Private sector spending includes money spent on health care providers other than doctors (chiropractors and naturopaths, for example); institutions other than hospitals (nursing homes and so on); and pharmaceuticals, dental care, eye care, and private insurance premiums (to cover such expenses as medication, dental, and eye care). In Alberta and British Columbia, people must also pay premiums for public health care, the rate of which is determined by one's income (ability to pay).

202 * BETTER MEDICINE

The United States

There are two major government funded health insurance programs in the United States: Medicare, which covers elderly Americans (aged sixty-five and over) and disabled Americans, and Medicaid, which provides health insurance and services for lower-income Americans. Both programs came into being in the mid-1960s and currently cover almost 27 percent of the American population.

Medicare is a federal program that reimburses the elderly for their health care expenses. In the senior population, 98.6 percent are enrolled in Medicare and most elderly (70 percent) have both Medicare and additional private insurance for those costs not covered by the public program (there are estimates that Medicare only covers half of the health care costs of its beneficiaries).[8] Medicaid is a joint federal-state program and therefore its benefits and eligibility requirements vary from state to state. In 1997, Medicare covered 38.4 million Americans and Medicaid had 33.6 million recipients.[9]

The federal government spends its health care dollars on these programs (which cover at least a portion of the cost of hospital, nursing home, medication, physician care, and other expenses), as well as funding research and development, veterans' care, etc. State governments contribute to Medicaid, and also fund such things as public health services, community-based services (mental health and substance abuse services, for example), state university-based teaching hospitals, state employee health premiums, etc.

In 1997, the public sector in the United States accounted for 46.4 percent of total health care spending; the private sector comprised 53.6 percent.[10]

There are various types of private insurance offered in the United States, including fee-for-service plans, managed care (health maintenance organizations [HMOs], preferred provider organizations, and the like), and recently, medical savings accounts (MSAs). About 70 percent of Americans have private insurance, most of which is obtained through employment.[11]

Health insurance is not mandatory in the United States and about 43.4 million Americans were uninsured in 1997 (16.1 percent of the population).[12] But being uninsured in the United States does not mean that a person will not receive medical care if they require it. By law, neither public nor private hospitals are permitted to refuse treatment to an indigent patient. The 1986 Consolidated Omnibus Budget Reconciliation Act (COBRA) includes a section that addresses the problem of "patient dumping," which is the denial of care or the transfer of patients to another hospital based on ability to pay for care.[13]

The cost of health care was a major concern in the United States in the 1990s. This is one reason that managed care, which explicitly attempts to control costs, has proliferated in the United States. On the public sector front, there were estimates that both Medicare and Medicaid were set to go bankrupt if changes were not implemented. In 1997, the Balanced Budget Act (BBA) created the National Bipartisan Commission on the Future of Medicare. It has been charged with examining the Medicare program and making recommendations on financing health care for the elderly and the disabled in the twenty-first century.

The incremental reforms expected to result from the BBA include a slowing of the growth in annual per capita Medicare costs (to be achieved by tightening prospective payment rates to health care providers, hospitals, and managed care plans and by reducing benefits to certain beneficiaries). The reforms will also attempt to improve protections for low-income Medicare recipients (as there are several health care items that the program does not cover, such as prescription medications).

Germany

The foundations of the German health care system date back to 1883 and Chancellor von Bismarck. The main element of Bismarck's system remains in place today: statutory health insurance composed of competing sickness funds.

About 87 percent of the German population belong to the statutory health insurance (SHI) system. Sickness funds are decentralized, self-administered, nonprofit organizations and less than 10 percent of them are run by private insurance companies. Sickness funds are financed by equal contributions from employers and employees. The premiums are a fixed percentage of an employee's income and are not related to his or her age, sex, or health status. Unemployed individuals are covered by health insurance paid for by the government and it is estimated that only 0.1 percent of Germans have no health insurance at all.[14]

Those Germans with an income above a defined threshold are permitted to opt out of the public system and purchase private insurance; about 9 percent of Germans have chosen this option. Premiums for private health insurance are related to an individual's age, sex, and health status.[15]

Insurance companies have to accept everyone who applies, and there is a basic benefits package that the companies must offer. Insured persons are allowed to choose their own sickness fund and to change from one fund to another.[16] As well, insured people are permitted to choose their own physicians.

The federal government provides the regulatory framework for health care, but the *Lander* (provinces) are responsible for providing the care — they help fund hospitals, medical education, etc. Most hospitals are owned either by the *Lander*, local governments, or charities.

In each *Lander*, the regional associations of the sickness funds negotiate with the regional associations of primary care physicians, specialists, and hospitals to determine the fee schedule for care provided in a hospital setting. For insured persons, hospital care is almost free at the point of delivery; there is a minimal user fee. There are also fees for some services, such as eye care and dental care. Most ambulatory care is free at the point of delivery for insured persons and local public health offices provide social, psychiatric, and family services that are free to all. There are copayments required for pharmaceuticals and the government has a list of medications that it subsidizes.

In Germany, there has been a separation between hospital and primary health care. Prior to the 1993 Health Care Structure Act, primary care physicians were not permitted to treat patients in hospitals and hospitals could not provide outpatient surgeries or services. In addition, long-term care in Germany has been available in hospitals historically, but a law introduced in 1995 provided for long-term care insurance to support care at home provided by family members, neighbours, or home nurses.

The Reform Act of SHI 2000 became effective in January 2000. It aims to remove ineffective or unproven technologies and pharmaceuticals from the benefits package; increase cooperation among general practitioners, ambulatory specialists, and hospitals; and improve the funding mechanisms for physicians and hospitals.

Switzerland

Since 1996, it has been compulsory for Swiss citizens to have sickness insurance and an insurance company is prohibited from refusing anyone coverage. Even prior to the Compulsory Health Insurance Act, however, it was estimated that about 99 percent of the Swiss population was voluntarily insured against illness.[17]

The government does not provide health insurance; private companies do. Premiums are not linked to income but take into account age of entry into the plan, regional cost differences, and gender.[18] There is a basic set of benefits that insurers must cover by law and citizens who cannot afford the insurance premiums receive an income supplement (not a health premium subsidy) from the *canton* (province). The public sector — confederation, *cantons*, and districts — also provides subsidies for hospitals, long-term care, and home care.

Based on the required set of benefits that insurers must offer, insurers within each *canton* must pay a portion of their premiums into a regional fund. "The relative financial risk of each insurer is then calculated and insurers with a larger proportion of less healthy, high-risk members receive from the fund an amount that compensates adequately for the higher financial risks involved in insuring their members. In effect, the insurers with healthier members subsidize those with less healthy members."[19] Such a system helps to prevent insurers from skimming all of the healthy people from the population and leaving those who are less healthy either without coverage, with very expensive coverage, or needing to be looked after by the government.

There are various ways in which insurers contract with health care providers. Health maintenance organizations that buy pharmaceuticals and medical services for their members in large quantities provide an affordable insurance option for many Swiss. As well, some insurance companies have been discussing the introduction of bonuses that would be paid to patients if they use less than a specified amount of health services in a given period.[20]

According to Organisation of Economic Co-Operation and Development (OECD) data, public expenditures account for 69.3 percent of total health care spending in Switzerland, while the private sector accounts for 30.7 percent.

The United Kingdom

Established in 1948, the National Health Service (NHS) is the main provider of health care in the United Kingdom. It has provided the model for many socialized health care systems; it is based on the ideal of universal coverage for all British citizens, paid for from general tax revenues.

The scope of the NHS has narrowed since its inception — dental care, eye care, and prescription charges, for example, are not covered any longer — and there always has been a private system in the U.K., which operates parallel to the public system (providing acute, long-term, and other types of care). While the NHS insures everyone, people are permitted to buy insurance and/or any medical service from private suppliers. About 11 percent of the U.K. population has private medical insurance, although some private patients do not have insurance and pay directly when they need treatment.[21]

The most fundamental changes to the U.K. health system came in the last decade. The reforms of the early 1990s introduced an "internal market" into the NHS. There were three main components in this effort to inject more choice and competition into the public system: the creation of general practice fundholding schemes, the establishment of NHS trusts, and the creation of a purchaser-provider split.

General practitioners (GPs) were given the option of becoming *fundholders*. These fundholding practices of one or more GPs not only provided general medical services, but were also given an additional sum of money with which to purchase, on behalf of their patients, certain services (mainly elective surgery) from their choice of provider. Prior to 1990, such decisions were made by a health authority (public bodies that operated health care services for given geographical populations within budgets provided by the central government).

As well, NHS *trusts* were established. These semiautonomous bodies were established to assume responsibility for the ownership and management of hospitals or other facilities previously managed or provided by a health authority, or to manage and provide new hospitals and other facilities within the public sector.[22]

The *purchaser-provider split* created a clear demarcation between the providers of a service (the NHS trusts) and the purchasers of that service (the health authorities and the GP fundholders on behalf of their patients). All NHS hospitals were run by NHS trusts; they received no money directly from the government, but instead obtained orders for their services from the purchasers. The "internal market" required providers to compete with each other — on the basis of quality and price — to attract purchasers who were permitted to contract with providers outside their regions.

The 1999 Health Act abolished GP fundholding and replaced it with primary care groups, which will eventually become primary care trusts (PCTs). PCTs will include GPs, other health professionals, social services, and members of the local community. They will be corporate bodies with their own budgets for the health care of their population — at least 100,000 people per trust.

Other changes enacted by the 1999 legislation allow for additional payments to health authorities based on their performance, increase the ability of the government to control the prices of and profits from pharmaceuticals, and steepen the penalties of defrauding the NHS. As well, the National Institute for Clinical Excellence has been established to appraise and provide guidance on the clinical and cost effectiveness of new and existing health technologies (including medications).

Among the reforms implemented in the 1990s was the development of a Patient's Charter in 1991. The charter specifies the standard of health care that a patient has the right to expect, which includes being given detailed information about local health services, quality standards, and maximum waiting times for treatment.

Australia[23]

The government accounts for 72 percent of health expenditures in Australia; its Medicare program provides access to medical and hospital services for all Australian residents. The legislation pertaining to the main elements of the program is contained in the 1993 Health Insurance Act.

Medicare benefits are based on fees determined for each medical service. Two levels of Medicare benefit are payable: for professional services provided in a hospital, the Medicare benefit is 75 percent of the schedule fee; for all other professional services, the Medicare benefit is generally 85 percent of the schedule fee. Thus, the 28 percent spent on health care by Australia's private sector is composed of out-of-pocket payments made by individuals for insurance premiums and care not covered by Medicare. People may insure privately for care in private hospitals, and people may insure with private insurance companies for the gap in the Medicare benefit and the schedule fee. The fee gap exists because the government has no legal power to control the rate doctors charge and can only restrict the amount that health funds (insurers) can reimburse patients to the Medicare benefits schedule.

Insurance premiums in Australia — public and private — are community rated. That is, health funds cannot discriminate against people by charging them differential premiums based on their risk (age, sex, health status, and lifestyle). People can switch between two health funds without penalty.

Last year, the federal government introduced Lifetime Health Cover in an effort to slow down the rate of premium increases and make private health insurance more affordable. The program takes into account the length of time that a person has had private hospital insurance and rewards them by offering lower premiums. For example, a thirty-year-old joining the program today will pay lower premiums throughout his or her years of membership than someone who first joins at fifty years of age.

As well, Australia has recently introduced the federal government's 30 percent rebate initiative. For every $1 that people contribute to their private health insurance premium, the government refunds 30¢.

The government is hopeful that the private sector will reduce pressure on public hospitals and public budgets. In other cost-related initiatives, Australia has tried to contain pharmaceutical expenses through measures such as patient cost sharing, generic drug incentives, and price negotiation with suppliers.[24]

Singapore

In Singapore, the delivery of health care is divided between the provision of primary care by private medical practitioners' clinics and government polyclinics, and secondary and tertiary specialist care in public and private hospitals. Patients can visit any provider in either system. Private practitioners provide about 80 percent of primary health care while the polyclinics provide the remaining 20 percent. For hospital care the situation is reversed, with the government providing 80 percent of the care and the private sector, 20 percent.[25] On the financing side, of total health care expenditures in 1998, government spending is about 31 percent and private sector (households and businesses) spending, 69 percent.

Patients are expected to pay at least part of the cost for the medical services they use, and to pay more if they demand higher levels of service in terms of comfort and amenities. In the government polyclinics, 50 percent of the cost for primary care is subsidized. In the public hospitals (the majority of which are restructured hospitals that have been incorporated as private companies, but are wholly owned by the government), patients can opt for different classes of ward accommodation, ranging from Class A (for which patients pay the full cost) to Class C (for which the government subsidizes 80 percent of the cost). Patients of all classes receive comparable levels of medical care and no Singaporean is denied access to the health care system or use of emergency services at public hospitals.[26]

Private hospitals are not required to accept all patients. In private hospitals and outpatient clinics, patients must pay the amount charged by the hospitals and doctors on a per-day or fee-for-service basis. Prices for medical care in the private sector are not regulated, but there are guidelines set by the doctors' representative body, the Singapore Medical Association. As well, the government-regulated public sector medical charges act as a benchmark for private sector providers.

There are private insurers in Singapore, but the government organizes the main methods of health funding and insurance. The government's philosophy is that people should be encouraged to adopt healthy lifestyles and be responsible for their own health. To this end, it has created three programs: Medisave, Medishield, and Medifund.

Medisave is not an insurance scheme but a compulsory savings plan to help pay for any hospitalization costs, especially after retirement. It is part of the country's Central Provident Fund (CPF), a fund into which both employees and employers contribute roughly the same amount for an employee's retirement, housing needs, and, since 1984, health care. It operates as a payroll tax and the health care portion amounts to 6 to 8 percent of an employee's salary, depending on his or her age group. The contributions are tax deductible and earn interest. Singaporeans can withdraw from their medical savings account to pay for their own hospital bills or bills of immediate family members. They keep any amount that remains in their account; it is transferred to the CPF ordinary account and can be used for purchasing any government-approved investments.

Medishield was introduced in July 1990 to supplement Medisave. It is a voluntary insurance plan designed to help Singaporeans meet any medical expenses that arise from a major accident or prolonged illness. Medishield premiums are paid from Medisave contributions.

Medifund is an endowment fund set up by the government as a safety net to help low-income citizens to pay for their medical care. Anyone who is unable to pay for even subsidized hospital care can apply for help from Medifund, which provides grants to certain hospitals and medical institutions.

South Africa

Health insurance is voluntary in South Africa, and the public system is available for those South Africans who cannot afford to pay for health care themselves or who are not members of an insurance plan. It is estimated that the public system is responsible for approximately 80 percent of the South African population and composes about 40 percent of total health care spending; the private sector, while covering about 20 percent of the population, accounts for almost 60 percent of the money spent on health care.[27]

Most public sector health funding goes toward acute care, with only 11 percent directed toward primary care. The private sector — households, employers, and insurance companies — also spends 11 percent of its resources on primary care, but directs larger portions of its funds to medicines (32 percent), private hospitals (18 percent), and hospital specialists (18 percent). The remainder of private funds is divided among dentists (10 percent), public hospitals (4 percent), and other/administration (7 percent).[28]

There are two categories of private insurance: not-for-profit medical aid schemes that are mainly available to employed South Africans, and for-profit insurance that is available to anyone who can afford it. Premiums for the medical aid schemes are based on income and the number of dependents, while premiums for the for-profit insurers are risk-rated by client or client group.

Various insurance companies offer different types of programs: some offer managed care schemes, and some offer medical savings account programs. Reforms being considered by the government with respect to the medical insurance market include the expansion of medical aid schemes (especially to older and sicker South Africans) by changing to a community-based risk-rating method, and the provision of a basic set of prescribed benefits.

As with financing, the delivery of health is shared by the public and private sectors. The majority of general practitioners (62 percent), medical specialists (77 percent), pharmacists (88 percent), and dentists (89 percent) work in the private sector; about half of the nurses and 31 percent of auxiliary staff work in the private sector.[29] Since 1997, medical, dental, and certain other health care professionals have had to do remunerated compulsory community service at state hospitals for one year, prior to being able to set up private practice.[30]

With respect to health facilities, there are public hospitals and clinics; private, not-for-profit facilities; and private, for-profit facilities. Public facilities are owned and operated by the government. Private, not-for-profit health facilities receive government funding but are operated by autonomous managers governed by committees or boards. The private, for-profit sector is made up of organizations that work outside the government's direct control (although they are regulated and can contract with governments to provide certain services to nonprivate patients).

Copayments are charged in public facilities for medical care, but there is no systematic collection system and many patients do not pay the fees. Health professionals in the public sector are salaried, while doctors in the private sector and private hospitals are paid fee-for-service (private sector nurses are salaried).

The responsibility for public health care is divided among the national, provincial, and local governments. While each level has numerous responsibilities — some of which overlap — the national government formulates policy and legislation and funds the other levels of government; the provinces plan for and provide mainly acute care; and the local authorities provide primary care.

There is debate about the potential of a national public insurance plan to resolve the existing inequities in the care being provided to public vs. private patients, urban vs. rural patients, and black vs. white patients. However, health care delivery is being reoriented to focus on primary health care based on a district health system model. The ideal district would be responsible for a population of between 50,000 and 500,000 — large enough to have a full range of health services, but small enough to promote community involvement in health care.[31] The idea is for districts to integrate all aspects of the health care system: make and implement policy decisions, organize and provide a range of preventive to curative/hospital care, provide public services, and contract for private provision of services. The reforms are not complete.

3. International Health Care Comparisons

Numerous international comparisons of health status and spending exist. The most commonly compared health status measures are life expectancy, mortality rates (overall, maternal, and infant), and fertility rates. The predominant spending measures are total, public, and private spending on health care as a percentage of a country's gross domestic product. In analyses of health care resources, physicians per capita, hospital beds per thousand population, and average length of in-patient stay (in days) are often considered.

These factors provide an idea of how well certain areas of a country's health care system perform relative to those in other countries. But what conclusions can be drawn from the fact that the United States spends more on health care than Canada or that Canadians have a longer life expectancy than Americans? Such one-variable measurements do not capture the complexities of an entire health care system. The World Health Organization's recent *World Health Report 2000: Health Systems: Improving Performance* is the only study that attempts to evaluate and rank the overall performance of health care systems worldwide.

WHO defines a health care system as being the provider of health services (preventive, curative, and palliative interventions). In its *World Health Report 2000*, WHO provides an index of national health system performance that shows how a particular country achieves three main goals: good health, responsiveness to the expectations of the population, and fairness of financial contribution. For good health, WHO examined disability-adjusted life years (life spent free of disability as opposed to life expectancy only); for responsiveness, a survey determined how patients are treated within the system (dignity, autonomy, confidentiality, promptness of service, etc.); and for fairness of financial contribution, WHO focused on how much people are required to pay for health care services out-of-pocket (with the assumption that less is better).

One WHO ranking shows how well the health care systems are reaching their potential. In this ranking of overall health system performance, the leaders are France, Italy, San Marino, Andorra, and Malta. Singapore places 6th in overall system performance, the United Kingdom 18th, Switzerland 20th, Germany 25th, Canada 30th, Australia 32nd, the United States 37th, and South Africa 175th out of 191 countries.

While the WHO ranking is an important contribution to the evaluation of health care system performance, WHO advocates for all countries — developed and developing — a health system that encompasses everything from road safety to prevention to surgery. WHO would like such a system to be universally accessible, with more public financing, insurance, and coordination for health care. For WHO, "the ideal is largely to disconnect a household's financial contribution to the health care system from its health risks, and separate it almost entirely from the use of needed services."[32]

While WHO concludes that out-of-pocket payment for and private financing of health care are unfair and should be reduced, the study discussed in the next section attempts to remain neutral on this point. Rather than looking at the "fairness" of financing, it looks at the fairness of the care provided to various groups in the population by examining the differences in health status between low- and high-income regions, and majority and minority populations.

4. An Eight-Country Study of Health System Performance

The study discussed in this section provides an alternative to the WHO method of ranking health care systems. It makes no a priori assumptions as to whether a public or private health care system is preferable. It examines the financing and delivery of health care in eight countries — Canada, the United States, Germany, Switzerland, the United Kingdom, Australia, Singapore, and South Africa — and attempts to determine if any of these countries has a health system that is significantly more efficient and effective at providing care and improving population health.

For the most part, the data used in this index come from the OECD, the WHO, the World Bank, the United Nations, and each country's health department/ministry. The decision of how to rank country performance is based on the paradigm of what should constitute a health care system's principles when trying to achieve better health status for a population: high-quality care, broad access to care, and low costs.

Data were collected for some 100 variables (from life expectancy to the number of hospital beds per capita to the amount of out-of-pocket spending on health care), which are grouped into the following 17 larger categories: demographics, socioeconomic status, health status, mortality rates, preventable illnesses, health coverage, equality, distribution of health spending, availability of services, technology, appropriateness of services, patient satisfaction, efficiency, sustainability, total health spending, public and private sector spending.[33]

Quality of care is measured using the categories of health status, mortality rates, preventable illnesses, appropriateness of services, and patient satisfaction. Access to care takes into account the amount of insurance coverage in a population, equity in health outcomes, how health spending is distributed between acute and other health care services, and the availability of medical expertise and technology. Cost considers efficiency and total health spending, as well as sustainability.

The index used in the study is calculated in the same way as the UN Human Development Index and the Fraser Institute Index of Human Progress (see Appendix II).[34] It shows how one health care system performs relative to another. The scores range from 0 to 100, and a higher index score indicates better health system performance. These scores are summarized in Table 1.

Results

Quality of Care

Canada ranks first in health status. This category includes life expectancy, healthy (free-of-disability) life expectancy, the percent of population not expected to survive to age forty, self-reported health status, and the prevalence of smoking, alcohol consumption, and obesity in the population.

Singapore, however, has the lowest mortality rates. And the United Kingdom ranks highest in the categories of preventable illnesses (with relatively low rates of tuberculosis, HIV infection, etc.) and appropriateness of services (with relatively low rates of C-sections and medications consumed per capita, two indicators of the appropriateness of medical care).

Switzerland has the highest patient satisfaction, due to short waiting times for nonemergency treatment and a high system-responsiveness ranking given by the WHO in *World Health Report 2000*. The WHO score is based on the performance of a country's health system regarding patient dignity, autonomy and confidentiality, prompt attention, quality of basic amenities, access to social support networks during care, and choice of health care provider.

Access to Care

In Switzerland, health insurance is mandatory, and in Canada, the United Kingdom, and Australia, every citizen is eligible for health insurance provided by the public sector. These countries, therefore, rank highly in terms of health coverage. Canada and the United Kingdom also share relatively high immunization rates, which is an indication of citizen's access to basic public health services.

Data on care equality were not readily available. This study includes, however, data on the differences in life expectancy, infant mortality, and low birth weight between high- and low-income regions, and majority and minority populations in South Africa, Canada, the United States, Australia, and Singapore. Of these countries, Singapore ranks highest, with the minority Indian population possessing an infant mortality rate that is 2.4 births per 1,000, which is higher than that of the majority Chinese population. At the other extreme is Australia, where the difference in infant mortality rate is 10.2 births per 1,000 between the general and indigenous populations.

Regarding the distribution of health care spending, the United States directs the largest proportion of health spending to prevention and public health, but all eight countries spend most of their health care dollars on acute care and pharmaceuticals.

With respect to the availability of health care resources, Germany ranks first with more hospital beds per person and more physicians, specialists, and dentists per 1,000 population than the other countries. While Switzerland comes second to Australia with respect to computed tomography (CT) scans and second to the United States with respect to magnetic resonance imagers (MRIs), it attains the top ranking in the technology category.

Cost of Care

While there is some debate as to whether high health care spending is positive or negative, the traditional perspective is that health costs must be contained. Therefore, this study assumes that more spending on health is worse than less. Thus, both Singapore and South Africa rank highly, while the United States receives a score of zero for this category.

The sustainability of a health care system is dependent on whether a country can afford to maintain it. The projected percentage of the population over sixty-five years old and the amount spent on them relative to the rest of the population are included in this category. Sustainability also includes the number of medical students, expenditure on research and development (R&D), and the number of R&D scientists and technicians. Switzerland is in the most favourable position regarding the future of its health system; the United States and Australia, the worst.

Overall Country Rankings

The overall score is an average of all the category scores excluding demographics, socioeconomic status, public sector spending, and private sector spending. The demographics and socioeconomic status groups are not included in the calculation because a country's health care system is not responsible for shaping these conditions; rather, it must operate under these conditions. Neither public nor private sector spending is included in the overall score in Table 1 because there is no consensus on which form of financing is more efficient and effective.

Overall, Singapore ranks highest, followed by the United Kingdom, Switzerland, Germany, Australia, Canada, the United States, and South Africa. The *World Health Report 2000* yields a similar ranking, even though it uses a different methodology. The only difference is that the order of Australia and Canada is reversed in the WHO study, with Canada ranking higher than Australia.

Table 2 provides four separate rankings of the eight countries' overall scores. The first ranking simply arranges the overall scores from Table 1 from highest to lowest. The second ranking is based on the assumption that public sector spending is the "better" method of financing a health care system, the third assumes that private sector spending is "better," and the fourth takes spending out of the index entirely.

The public ranking puts the United Kingdom first, followed by Switzerland, Germany, Canada, Singapore, Australia, the United States, and South Africa. Singapore regains its first-place standing in the private ranking and Australia moves to second place, followed by Germany, the United States, Switzerland, Canada, the United Kingdom, and South Africa. If the amount spent on health (total, public, or private) is not included in the index at all, then Germany places first, followed by Switzerland, the United Kingdom, Singapore, the United States, Canada, Australia, and South Africa.

5. Conclusions

Contrary to the common belief in Canada, the health index scores demonstrate that either a publicly or privately funded health care system can deliver timely, quality medical care to all citizens. First-place Singapore (overall ranking) relies heavily on private sector financing for health care and puts much responsibility on patients to finance at least a portion of the cost of their care. Second-place United Kingdom (overall ranking) possesses a private system that operates alongside its National Health Service.

As well, Canada is not the only country in the world that values universality. In terms of access to care, *all eight* countries have measures that attempt to ensure that their citizens receive health care when they need it, regardless of their ability to pay. Conversely, no system has successfully eliminated inequalities in health status across socioeconomic or racial groups. Canada, Australia, the United States, and South Africa exhibit significant inequalities in health status. There is minimal data for Singapore and no data for Germany, Switzerland, and the United Kingdom on this aspect of health care delivery.

As with most studies of this nature, the main conclusion is that more and higher-quality data are needed. A well-defined set of performance indicators would help policy-makers, funders, and health managers in the management of health care systems and policy development. It would help patients better monitor the quality of the system into which their tax dollars are going and from which they must receive their health care. It would also facilitate more in-depth analysis among countries, allowing a country to more readily adopt into its own health care system elements of another country's system that seem to be particularly effective at improving health.

TABLE 1

Summary of Health Index Scores

(Score: 100 = best/most, 0 = worst/least)

	South Africa (SA)	Canada (CA)	United States (US)	Germany (GR)	Switzerland (SW)	United Kingdom (UK)	Australia (AU)	Singapore (SG)	Highest Scorer
Demographics	60.0	46.0	28.2	52.2	46.2	32.0	49.2	70.4	SG
Socioeconomic Status	3.7	68.3	71.5	52.7	65.4	58.0	58.5	57.5	US
Health Status	23.5	82.7	66.9	72.5	73.4	62.6	63.4	80.1	CA
Mortality Rates	30.8	70.1	64.2	67.9	70.3	67.8	70.6	70.8	SG
Preventable Illnesses	22.6	75.6	71.4	89.8	81.9	94.9	87.0	90.9	UK
Health Coverage	23.3	88.0	32.7	62.6	100.0	95.5	86.7	40.2	SW
Equality	16.8	85.9	63.5	. . .	. . .	. . .	33.3	100.0	SG
Distribution of Health Spending	97.8	41.0	39.8	39.6	12.7	50.8	23.3	0.0	SA
Availability of Services	17.7	48.9	54.5	76.6	68.6	35.4	50.2	16.3	GR
Technology	. . .	6.2	74.5	74.7	88.3	14.2	60.0	. . .	SW
Appropriateness of Services	. . .	52.2	79.1	44.0	0.0	85.2	71.6	. . .	UK
Patient Satisfaction	43.0	27.9	45.7	63.6	88.0	41.0	47.9	49.1	SW
Efficiency	86.7	64.4	69.1	41.5	34.7	53.5	40.3	94.5	SG
Sustainability	50.0	37.7	35.7	40.0	54.9	47.7	35.7	46.8	SW
Total Health Spending	87.4	56.8	0.0	34.6	37.3	77.8	68.2	94.7	SG
Public Sector Spending	31.6	38.3	24.2	76.2	78.4	89.9	32.4	18.9	UK
Private Sector Spending	49.6	15.9	66.2	55.5	30.3	3.9	61.8	59.5	US
Overall Score*	45.4	56.7	53.6	59.0	59.2	60.5	56.8	62.1	SG

* Overall score does not include demographics, socioeconomic status, public sector spending, and private sector spending. The variables used to calculate the scores and the individual indicator scores within each group appear in Appendix I.

TABLE 2

Ranking of Health Care Systems from "Best" to "Worst"

Overall ranking*: Indifferent to public and private sector funding

1	Singapore	62.1
2	United Kingdom	60.5
3	Switzerland	59.2
4	Germany	59.0
5	Australia	56.8
6	Canada	56.7
7	United States	53.6
8	South Africa	45.4

Public ranking**: Public sector is preferred funder of health care

1	United Kingdom	65.2
2	Switzerland	61.3
3	Germany	59.1
4	Canada	57.3
5	Singapore	57.1
6	Australia	53.9
7	United States	50.3
8	South Africa	44.7

Private ranking**: Private sector is preferred funder of health care

1	Singapore	63.4
2	Australia	57.8
3	Germany	56.2
4	United States	55.9
5	Switzerland	54.4
6	Canada	54.3
7	United Kingdom	52.9
8	South Africa	47.5

No health spending**: Total, public, and private sector spending excluded

1	Germany	61.2
2	Switzerland	61.1
3	United Kingdom	59.0
4	Singapore	58.9
5	United States	58.1
6	Canada	56.7
7	Australia	55.8
8	South Africa	41.2

* Overall ranking does not include demographics, socioeconomic status, public sector spending, or private sector spending.
** Public, private, and no health spending rankings do not include demographics and socioeconomic status.

Appendix I

Variables included in the calculation of the eight-country health care system performance index:

Demographics

Total population: current size and annual growth rate
Dependency ratio (population under age 15 and over age 65 as a percentage of the population aged 15–64)
Percentage of population aged 65 years and older
Total fertility rate (live births per woman)

Socioeconomic Status

United Nations Human Development Index ranking
Fraser Institute Human Progress Index ranking
Average years of education for population aged 25 and older
Literacy rate (percentage of population)
Labour force (percentage of population)
Unemployment rate (percentage of population)
Wage and salaried employment (mean earnings in purchase power parity [PPP] dollars)
Percentage of population with low income (definition of low income varies between countries)
Percentage of population living under U.S.$1 per day
Real GDP per capita in 1997 (U.S.$)
GNP per capita (annual growth rate)

Health Status

Life expectancy at birth (years)
Health expectancy at birth (years)
People not expected to survive to age 40 (percentage of total population)
Perceived health (good/very good health as a percentage of the population)
Smokers (percentage of population)
Cigarettes per smoker per year
Alcohol (percentage of drinkers in the population)
Obesity (percentage of population with body mass index >30 kg/m2)
Potential years of life lost (PYLL) prior to age 70, per 100,000 population

Mortality Rates

Mortality rate, all causes (per 100,000 population)
Infant mortality rate (per 1,000 live births)
Probability of dying under age 5 (per 1,000 population)
Probability of dying, ages 15–59 (per 1,000 population)
Maternal mortality ratio (per 100,000 population)

Preventable Illnesses

Low birth weight (percentage of total live births)
Spina bifida (rate per 10,000 births)
Prevalence of HIV (percentage of adults)
AIDS cases per 1,000 population
Tuberculosis per 100,000 population

Health Coverage

Children immunized against measles (percentage of children under 12 months)

Children immunized: diptheria, tetanus, pertussis (percentage of children under 12 months)

Women reporting having had at least one mammogram (percentage of age group)

Minimum population with or required to have insurance for health care (percentage of population)

Percentage of population eligible for public insurance/required to have insurance for acute care

Percentage of population eligible for public insurance/required to have insurance for outpatient care

Percentage of population eligible for public insurance/required to have insurance for medications

Percentage of population eligible for public insurance/required to have insurance for therapeutic devices

Equality

Difference in life expectancy between majority and identifiable minority populations

Difference in life expectancy between high- and low-income regions

Difference in infant mortality between majority and identifiable minority populations

Difference in infant mortality between high- and low-income regions

Difference in low birth weight between majority and identifiable minority populations

Difference in low birth weight between high- and low-income regions

Difference in percentage of population uninsured between majority and identifiable minority populations

Difference in percentage of population uninsured between high- and low-income regions

Distribution of Health Spending

Total acute care expenditures as percentage of total health expenditures

Total expenditure on prevention and public health as percentage of total health expenditures

Total expenditure on pharmaceuticals as percentage of total health expenditures

Availability of Health Care Services

Inpatient care beds per 1,000 population

Acute care beds per 1,000 population

Psychiatric beds per 1,000 population

Nursing home beds per 1,000 population

Percentage of births attended by skilled health staff

Coronary bypass operations per 100,000 population

Percentage of population using any type of alternative health care

Total health employment per 1,000 population

Practising physicians per 1,000 population

Practising specialists per 1,000 population

Practising certified/registered nurses per 1,000 population

Practising pharmacists per 1,000 population

Practising dentists per 1,000 population

Practising midwives per 1,000 population

Technology

Magnetic resonance imagers (MRIs) per million population
Computed tomography (CT) scanners per million population

Appropriateness of Services

Caesarian sections per 100,000 females
Medicines consumed per capita

Patient Satisfaction

World Health Organization system responsiveness ranking
Percentage of consumers/patients who believe minor changes to the health care system are needed
Percentage of consumers/patients who believe major changes to the health care system are needed
Percentage of consumers/patients who find physician care to be good/excellent
Percentage of consumers/patients who find hospital care to be good/excellent
Percentage of consumers/patients who waited less than one month for nonemergency treatment

Efficiency

Inpatient hospital days per capita
Percentage of population with in-patient admissions
Average lengths of stay (in-patient)
Average number of full-time-equivalent hospital employees per bed (acute care)
Physician consultations per capita

Sustainability

Medical enrollment/medical school students (per million population)
Total expenditure on health research and development (R&D) per capita ($PPP)
Expenditure on health R&D as percentage of GDP
R&D scientists and technicians per 1,000 population
Expenditure on 65-plus age group/expenditure for 0–64 group
Projected population 65-plus for 2015 as percentage population

Total Health Spending

Health care expenditures as a percentage of GDP
Total per capita health expenditures ($PPP)
Hospital expenditures per day ($U.S.)

Public Health Sector Spending

Public sector health spending as a percentage of GDP
Public sector health spending as a percentage of total health expenditures
Public expenditure on program administration and insurance (percentage of total health expenditures)
Public expenditure on home care (percentage of total health expenditures)
Public expenditure on pharmaceutical goods (percentage of total health expenditures)
Cost sharing (public/total) for total health care
Cost sharing (public/total) for in-patient acute care

Cost sharing (public/total) for outpatient care
Cost sharing (public/total) for pharmaceutical goods
Cost sharing (public/total) for therapeutic devices

Private Health Sector Spending

Private sector health spending as a percentage of total health expenditures
Private out-of-pocket spending on health care as a percentage of total health
expenditures
Private hospital beds per 1,000 population
Private hospital beds as a percentage of total bed stock

Appendix II

The health index used in this study is based on the UN Human Development Index and the Fraser Institute Index of Human Progress (Appendix I shows all of the variables used in the calculation of the index). It takes the following form when a higher value of an indicator is considered to be better than a lower value (higher life expectancy, more hospital beds, etc., positively affect health system performance):

$$\text{Index}_{Max=B} = [(\text{country} - \text{minimum}) \div (\text{maximum} - \text{minimum})] \times 100$$

In the equation, "country" is the observed value of a country for a particular indicator, "maximum" is the highest ranking of the eight countries for a particular indicator, and "minimum" is the lowest. $\text{Index}_{Max=B}$, then, is the index ranking when the higher (maximum) value is the "best."

In order for a higher index score to always indicate better health system performance, the index equation changes. $\text{Index}_{Max=W}$ is the index ranking when the higher value of an indicator is considered to be worse than a higher value (higher mortality rates, more people infected with HIV, more employees per hospital bed, etc., negatively affect health system performance):

$$\text{Index}_{Max=W} = [(\text{country} - \text{maximum}) \div (\text{minimum} - \text{maximum})] \times 100$$

For example, take the dependency ratio indicator (part of the demographics category); it is the number of people under 15 years old and over 64 years old expressed as a percentage of the population aged 15–64. A high dependency ratio means that there are many people the working population must support with their time and/or income. The country with the highest dependency ratio, therefore, is in the least desirable position relative to the other countries and receives the lowest score — a 0 — out of a possible 100 "points." The other countries receive values in between, depending on how close their dependency ratio is to that of the "worst" country.

In this case, Singapore receives a score of 100 because it has the lowest dependency ratio (41 percent); South Africa has the highest ratio (63 percent) and scores a 0. Germany, with a dependency ratio of 46.6 percent, receives the following score:

$$\text{Index}_{Max=W} = [(46.6 - 63) \div (41 - 63)] \times 100 = 75$$

Several indicators (and their index scores) form each of the larger categories mentioned previously: demographics, socioeconomic status, health status, etc. The category scores are averages of the indicator scores within the group. Singapore has the most favourable demographic situation, but because the category score is an average of all the indicators' scores, it receives a 70.4 on the demographics index — it was not the best country for every indicator.

NOTES

1. The 2001 Speech from the Throne, delivered by Governor General Adrienne Clarkson in the House of Commons, 30 Jan. 2001.
2. Speaking notes for Minister of Health Allan Rock, the Commonwealth Fund presentation in Washington, DC, 11 Oct. 2000. See the Health Canada Web site, www.hc-sc.gc.ca.
3. Canada Health Act Annual Report, 1999–2000 (Ottawa: Minister of Public Works and Government Services Canada, 2000), i.
4. Karen Donelan, Robert J. Blendon, Cathy Schoen, Karen Davis, and Katherine Binns, "The Cost of Health System Change: Public Discontent in Five Nations," Health Affairs, 18 (1999): 206–16.
5. "Canada's Prized Health-Care System in Crisis," Reuters, 13 Jan. 2000. See www.foxnews.com.
6. Michael Rachlis, Robert Evans, Patrick Lewis, and Morris Barer, Revitalizing Medicare: Shared Problems, Public Solutions (Vancouver: Tommy Douglas Research Institute, 2001), iii, 47.
7. Canadian Institute for Health Information, National Health Expenditure Trends, 1975–1999 (Ottawa: CIHI, 2000), 6.
8. Brian Biles, Susan Raetzman, Susan Joseph, and Karen Davis, "The Future of Medicare," Issue Brief (New York: Commonwealth Fund, 1998), 3.
9. U.S. Department of Health and Human Services, Health, United States, 1999 (Maryland: DHHS, 1999), 307–09.
10. Ibid., 284.
11. Ibid., 13.
12. Ibid., 319.
13. For more information on COBRA, see www.medlaw.com/.
14. Edward Griese, Christian Molt, Klaus-Jurgen Preuss, and Christoph Straub, "Germany: Private Health Sector Investment — Opportunities and Obstacles," session at the Fifth Annual International Summit on the Private Health Sector, Miami Beach, FL, 3–6 Dec. 2000.
15. Ibid.
16. World Health Organization Regional Office (Europe), Highlights on Health in Germany (Geneva: WHO, 1999), 38.
17. Paul Belien, "Patient Empowerment in Europe," Fraser Forum, Feb. 1998, 12–18.
18. Ibid.
19. Ibid.
20. Ibid.
21. See the section on private medicine in the U.K. at www.nhatoz.org.
22. Health Act 1999 (London: The Stationery Office, 1999).
23. The information in this section is taken from the Australian Department of Health and Aged Care Web site unless noted otherwise. See www.health.gov.au/.
24. Karen Davis, "International Health Policy: Common Problems, Alternative Strategies," Health Affairs 18.3 (May/June 1999): 138.
25. Singapore Ministry of Health Web site, www.gov.sg/moh/.
26. Ibid.
27. Health Systems Trust, South African Health Review 1999 (South Africa: HST, 2000), 70.

28. National Economic Research Associates, *The Health Care System in South Africa* (London: NERA, 1996), 26.

29. HST, *South African Health Review 1999*, 72.

30. South African government Web site, www.health.gov.za.

31. HST, *South African Health Review 1999*, 132.

32. World Health Organization, *The World Health Report 2000: Health Systems: Improving Performance* (Geneva: WHO, 2000).

33. See Appendix I for a detailed list of what variables are included in the 17 categories.

34. United Nations Development Programme, *The Human Development Report CD-ROM* (New York: UN Development Office Publications, 1999) and Joel Emes and Tony Hahn, "Measuring Development: An Index of Human Progress," *Public Policy Sources*, 36 (2000). See Appendix II for the detailed index equation.

PART 5

UP FROM STALEMATE

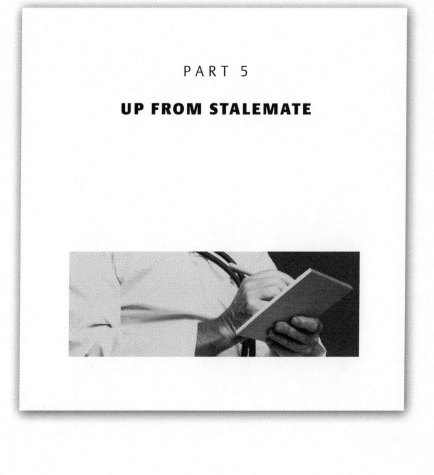

THIRTY-MILLION-TIER IS NEAR

William Watson

Discussions about health care rarely involve economics. That's not surprising, as many of Canada's most prominent health economists argue that economic principles don't readily apply to health issues; they argue that health care is a "market failure." In this animated consideration of economic principles and health care, economist William Watson discusses market failures and health care reforms.

Health care is more than public policy — it's personal. Drawing on his own experiences, Watson begins the essay by contemplating his "medicare epiphany" and outlines the positives and negatives of his experience. Extrapolating to the public at large, Watson notes that "... in proposing market-based reforms to medicare, it is important to understand that, in most Canadians' minds, free, universal health care does satisfy a significant moral imperative. It may not be why the system came into being — self-interest and *realpolitik* may have had much to do with that. . . . [I]t does explain why such a large proportion of Canadians evidently support the system. In their view, it is morally important that a lack of money not determine whether a person, especially a child, gets health care. Market-based reforms, if they are to succeed, must address that imperative."

Watson considers the importance of price in an economy. "Economics doesn't have many laws, but one it does have is that if you reduce a good's price, people will buy more of it." This law has implications for supply: generally, the lower the price, the lower the supply. Of course, medicare may provide health care to patients without direct cost, but prices are very much a part of the system, even if they are "administered" prices. Notes Watson, "The two main problems with 'administered' prices of this sort are . . . they can be wrong and they can be hard to change." Watson goes on to illustrate his argument by comparing public and market "price vectors."

While not perfect, there is an alternative to administered prices: the market. "Fans of the free market, like myself, often compare it with a never-ending referendum. People vote with their dollars and they never stop voting. They vote around the clock, all through the calendar. The market responds, not quite instantaneously but usually close enough, to their slightest commercial whim."

Most reform ideas, however, aren't built on the notion of free market principles. Indeed, the most popular ideas today focus on managing physician care (i.e., capitation-based payment) or adding financial resources (i.e., more funding). Watson rejects both ideas, calling for free market–based reforms. Such a concept may not be popular today, but Watson concludes with the following observation: "[A]s waiting lines lengthen, populations age, providers' unions grow stronger and more aggressive, and health care technology continues to be reinvented, we may be reaching the point where Canadian public opinion comes to accept that a private system with guarantees for the poor is less imperfect than a public system providing nominally equal, but slow and mediocre care."

Every Canadian has a medicare epiphany. Mine took place in the early 1990s in a waiting room of the Royal Victoria Hospital in Montreal. "The Vic" was built in what we used to call "the last century" (that is, the nineteenth) on the slopes of Mount Royal, so as to provide its patients with cleansing fresh air, verdant mountain walks, and inspiring views.

The waiting room was (what else would you expect?) hospital green. The chairs were plastic, the overhead lights fluorescent, the magazines ancient and no doubt germ-laden. The only decoration came in the form of charts of various kinds bearing advice for pregnant mothers and showing cutaway views of babies sleeping peacefully in wombs. My wife and I were there — in the usual cattle call of multiple appointments all made for the same hour, first come, first served — for her ultrasound examination. She was in her late thirties and having her first pregnancy, which meant an ultrasound was indicated. We queued with perhaps twenty other couples and single women. They were of several races and judging by their dress (admittedly a dangerous thing for a dishevelled university professor to do), from all classes. A number spoke languages I did not recognize.

As the minutes ticked by, it struck me this was the archetypal medicare experience:

- It was perfectly democratic: all were served. But everyone waited (unless friends, relatives, and special patients had been let in earlier. How would we have known?).
- The service was being rationed: not everyone who wanted an ultrasound got the test.
- Access was inconvenient: we had to go to a hospital halfway up a mountain to get it.
- The service itself was on the bubble: The Vic's ultrasound unit was in danger of closing because of budget cuts.
- The unit was subject to creeping privatization: if we wanted prints of the ultrasound image — which, of course, we did, as they represented the first glimpses of our child — we had to pay extra.

There it was, the good and the bad of medicare, all in one visit. The good was that no one was excluded. We upper-middle-class university professors were thrown in with people we normally wouldn't bump into in life (and wouldn't again, judging by the fact that most of the immigrants, having quickly acquired Canadian reserve, didn't converse). The bad was that we had to wait and that the service was inconvenient. It was not incompetent or especially unfriendly, though competence is hard to judge and it wasn't overly friendly. But it was inconvenient: friends of ours in New York who went through their first pregnancy at the same time reported that their doctor had an ultrasound machine in her office and an examination was routine for everyone. I don't know if their pictures were free.

As I sat in the waiting room I naturally thought about whether our baby was healthy, what the exam would be like and — a subject that preoccupied me at the time — becoming a father. But I also thought about medicare. (I'm an economist, and there was ample time for thought.) One thing I thought about was just what it is that we Canadians want out of medicare. One possibility is that we want free and perfectly equal access to medical services. If so, The Vic's waiting room was a pretty good microcosm of the system at large. It would give us democratic equality, though at a cost in the quality of service (for reasons that may be obvious, but which I'll nevertheless describe later).

Another possibility is that what Canadians want is a safety net. The nightmare people fear is that a devastating illness or accident will cause them to be wiped out financially: they'll lose their houses and their savings

in order to pay their hospital bills — if they get treatment, that is, for another concern is that, with a free market health care system, people in dire
need may simply be turned away for want of money, as (popular belief has
it) often happens in the United States. Of course, people increasingly are
denied service in Canada, too, and also for want of money — there is no
budget — but then the debate devolves to whether denying people service
is morally superior if it is done on the basis of wealth or according to more
random criteria. (Whether people actually are turned away in the U.S. as
often as Canadians think is an interesting factual question whose answer is
unlikely to alter the Canadian debate. *Ottawa Citizen* columnist John
Robson once pointed out that the infamous John Bobbitt, who suffered an
involuntary penile amputation at the hands of his enraged wife, had his
body part reconnected — in what presumably was an intricate and expensive operation — despite not having health insurance.[1])

These two possibilities — perfect egalitarianism versus a safety net —
figure prominently in the Canadian imagination of medicare. At a moral
level, they are compelling. Sitting in the waiting room of The Vic, in the
emotionally vulnerable psychological state I have since learned is typical of
imminent fatherhood, I had some inkling of how wrenching it would be
not to have access to the care that might let my son or daughter be born
and brought up free of disease or disability.

In that respect, health care *is* different. I feel no such inklings when wan-
dering through a Future Shop looking at home appliances that other,
poorer Canadians could not or should not (even if credit card companies
give them the money) consider buying. But the thought of a father or
mother seeing his or her child dying or suffering pain or disability because
they don't have enough money to pay for adequate health care is harrow-
ing to anyone not wholly incapable of empathy. The prospect of a family's
savings being wiped out by a disease their child might suffer should cause
similar empathy. So perhaps a third possibility should be added to the list:
maybe what Canadians really want is medicare for children, so that parents
never have to make a financial calculation when deciding whether to have
their child looked at by a physician.

A number of objections spring to mind, of course: people shouldn't have
children if they can't afford to care for them, whether pre- or postnatally.
And the answer to not being wiped out by ill health is good insurance,
which private carriers would be more than willing to provide at the right
price. If people can't afford good health insurance, the remedy may be to

provide them with money rather than free health care. As a pro-market conservative, I've made these arguments many times and doubtless will make them again. They are good arguments.

But in proposing market-based reforms to medicare, it is important to understand that, in most Canadians' minds, free, universal health care does satisfy a significant moral imperative. It may not be why the system came into being — self-interest and *realpolitik* may have had much to do with that. It may not explain why the system persists — the key players may have quite different motivations, including sunk emotional costs. But it does explain why such a large number of Canadians evidently support the system. In their view, it is morally important that a lack of money not determine whether a person, especially a child, gets care health. Market-based reforms, if they are to succeed, must address that imperative.

On the other hand, making sure that those without money get care does not require that everyone get exactly the same care for exactly the same price, and that that price be zero. We could have free care for poor people only. Or we could have free care for poor people and children. Or for poor people, children, and the aged — a combination the United States seems headed toward. Choosing instead to have free care for everyone on exactly the same basis has serious economic implications, which became increasingly clear through the 1990s.

What Prices Do

They had become clear for me in another medicare epiphany just months before my wife's ultrasound at The Vic. Sitting in my office, talking with a colleague on the telephone, I suffered a brief episode of aphasia (the inability to speak, an affliction that holds special terror for a university professor), followed by a severe headache. It was eventually diagnosed as classical migraine. It could, however, have been a ministroke.

The emergency care provided by medicare was actually quite good. The ambulance arrived at my office reasonably promptly. The reception team at (yes) The Vic was large, attentive, and very interventionist: they had my shirt off and electrodes attached to my chest virtually before I was through the door. But once I recovered from the immediate symptoms, which passed within minutes, the follow-up exams took six weeks. And they would have taken even longer except that my teaching schedule allowed me to set up camp outside the attending neurologist's office until someone cancelled and he could fit me into his schedule. Had I not had the luxury of a flexible work schedule, I assume it would have been even longer than a month and a half before I got a clean bill of circulatory health. As might be imagined, the six weeks that it took to do all the necessary tests — including a CT scan to rule out stroke as a diagnosis — were a period of considerable anxiety for a soon-to-be father. *Had* it been a stroke? Were strokes in my future? What would happen to my wife and child if I were to die or become disabled? Some people may be able to block such thoughts from their mind and sleep soundly while awaiting diagnostic tests. I suspect most of us can't. I certainly wouldn't. Some time later I learned from a visiting American economist that when he had suffered a similar aphasia, with what turned out to be the same diagnosis, his CT scan had been done the very next day. To avoid the anxiety of those six weeks, I would happily have paid a good deal of money.

(If I had a similar experience now, that trade-off would be possible. I could get diagnostics on short notice in exchange for money. In Quebec, most of the tests that were required are not classified as insured services when done outside hospitals, which means that private clinics operated after-hours by hospital staff are allowed to charge for them. Despite universal condemnation of the concept during the 2000 federal election, we already have two-tier health care: those with money can have their tests done quickly; those without must wait.)

That medicare should be slower than market-based care is hardly surprising. Economics doesn't have many laws, but one it does have is that if you reduce a good's price, people will buy more of it. There are exceptions — potatoes in nineteenth century Ireland, for instance. When their price fell people used the money they saved to cut back on potatoes and buy a scrap of meat instead. But that and similar exceptions are few enough to prove the rule. If people do not pay for their health care, they almost certainly will demand more of it than if they did have to balance the benefits they expect from care, including the alleviation of anxiety, against its financial cost.

True, it is sometimes argued that the demand for medicare services wouldn't respond to the price of such services and that user charges would therefore not reduce demand. That may be the case for some medical conditions: no one volunteers for a car crash just to get free reconstructive surgery. But many other medical services are taken up on a discretionary basis. With at least some visits to the doctor, people presumably are just on the margin of going or not going, and for many referred services, doctors presumably are just on the margin of referring or not referring. Charge a price and both patients and doctors may pull back from the margin.

There's a good deal of evidence that user charges or coinsurance payments do have this effect. The best-known study was conducted by the RAND think tank in the 1980s. It found that people who had to pay part of the cost of their care used less care, and that a coinsurance rate as low as 25 percent made a significant difference in demand. It also showed that "individuals with generous insurance buy more drugs." On the other hand, the rate at which people were admitted to hospitals did not differ by how much they had to pay, which suggests that in serious cases demand *is* "inelastic"; that is, not very responsive to price. A more recent study of the Kaiser Permanente HMO in northern California confirms that emergency department users who faced cash charges reduced their demand for services but that the reductions were greatest for the least serious complaints. Finally, in the early 1990s, a study of heart patients in King County, WA showed that people who faced copayments actually got to the hospital slightly faster after a myocardial infarction (a heart attack) than people who didn't. Financial considerations evidently do not cut demand when need is serious, but do when it is less so.

If data are not persuasive, however, there's always deduction. In fact, the belief that people *do* respond to price incentives is the usual rationale for eliminating prices from the system; we supposedly do not want people to take financial considerations into account when deciding whether or not to seek care. But if having to pay would lead them not to seek out service, it follows that free provision must increase demand.

It's not quite as clear what effect not charging for health services has on supply. In general, a higher price for a good or service — any good or service — will induce a greater supply of it. Granted, there are cases where greater supply simply can't be forthcoming: the number of Rembrandts, real Rembrandts at least, can only fall. There was only one Sinatra or Gretzky — increasing the price won't get you more. But the supply of health care, like the supply of most things, probably isn't perfectly "price-inelastic" in this way. Increasing its price probably will get you greater supply: more practitioners will work longer hours, fewer will leave the country, and more would-be practitioners will seek out training in the field or redouble their efforts to have credentials earned elsewhere recognized here. Supply may not increase overnight, but so long as entry into the "industry" is not blocked by regulation or custom, it will eventually increase.

By contrast, a lower price will generally reduce supply. If care were strictly free, if doctors received literally no remuneration for their services except the thanks of grateful patients and favourable consideration on Judgment Day, much less care would be provided than currently is. This is not to deny that many doctors provide at least some services *pro bono* or work longer hours than is sensible in light of their current remuneration, but simply to assert that, on average, they would likely do even more for higher pay.

In practice, of course, service isn't free: someone does pay, either an insurance company, workers' compensation, or a government. It's therefore hard to say whether not charging patients for medical service gets you more or less of it than if they did have to pay. It depends on how those in charge of the system decide to attract the supply that is then going to be given away free. Their choice may produce too much supply or too little. The health care system for federal politicians, who have access to Department of National Defence facilities, seems generously oversupplied. The health care system for the rest of us, which is characterized by longer and longer waits for more and more mediocre service, seems radically undersupplied. In fact, as a general rule, a planned system will probably create *both* too much and too little supply, producing shortages in some areas and surplus in others. I once heard a health official talk about how his province was "awash in urinalyses" — an evocative image, if ever there was one — because urinalyses had been priced too low for demanders and too high for suppliers, who made easy money performing them.

Whether the system gets supply "right" therefore depends on how whoever is in charge decides the services that are provided will be paid for. In our system, the responsible party is ultimately the minister of health. In fairness, most ministers of health probably learn very quickly that "the system" is harder to control than outsiders might imagine. Still, the minister does usually write most of the cheques that make the system work.

Critics of medicare commonly argue that it operates without prices and they/we therefore often draw analogies with Soviet Communism, analogies that — sometimes intentionally — infuriate the system's supporters. A good but bolshie (there we go again) friend of mine once exploded in rage when I referred to the system as "Stalinist." I had in mind medicare's frequent deliberate disregard for the information embodied in free-market prices, but he evidently assumed I was referring to something else (its indifferent approach to care, perhaps, or its monopoly over health resources, or its tendency to induce blind and intellectually ruthless obedience in its advocates). I have never seen him so incensed, though we have worked together on several projects that had high-pressure, stress-inducing deadlines.

In fact, Soviet Communism did use prices. They just weren't very informative prices. A colleague born and raised in the old Soviet Union tells of how prices were stamped into the handles of metal spoons. The possibility that spoon prices might actually change evidently was not considered.

The two main problems with "administered" prices of this sort are just that: they can be wrong and they can be hard to change. Wrong is not fatal. Free-market prices can be wrong, too. But their being wrong sets in train a sequence of events that corrects them. If people are lined up to buy a good or service, entrepreneurs soon notice and prices rise. In consequence, demand falls as consumers cut back and supply rises as new suppliers enter the market or old ones produce more. The upward pressure on price ends when demand and supply are equal. On the other hand, if goods are sitting on store shelves, then prices fall, causing producers to cut production and demanders to demand more, which once again brings demand and supply to equality, thus eliminating the glut. In both cases, demand and supply eventually meet and the price comes to rest until either costs or tastes change and another, also eventually self-correcting, imbalance occurs.

In a system of administered prices, on the other hand, prices that are too low don't rise unless the responsible minister allows them to. There is therefore no guarantee that shortages will be alleviated. The goods and services people want can't be found (except on the black market), but the price doesn't move unless the minister allows it to. And even if prices do rise, supply may not increase unless the minister allows more providers to enter the sector. The same is true for prices that are too high: the resulting excess supply will be cut, and deficient demand increased, only if the minister allows the price to fall.

Like a Soviet minister of production, a Canadian minister of health presides over a vast system of administered prices. The Canadian health sector is not nearly as large, either relatively or in absolute terms, as the Soviet economy was, but it represents a big chunk of Canadian economic activity (more than 6 percent of GDP) and it involves, at the very least, hundreds and hundreds of prices, some explicit, some implicit. What will physicians be paid for this or that service? How much in total will they be allowed to earn? How will hospitals, laboratories, and providers of other

238 • BETTER MEDICINE

ancillary services be compensated for the hundreds of things they do? Like the Soviet production minister, the Canadian health minister does not try to control all these prices on his or her own. The power to set a price is often decentralized, by delegation to a hospital or regional health board. But most such prices remain administered.

In theory at least, systems of administered prices need not be economically inefficient. Visiting China in the 1970s, John Kenneth Galbraith, an expert on the economics of price control (he helped run the U.S. Office of Price Administration during World War II) observed approvingly that the Chinese appeared to follow the rule that if demand exceeded supply and there were shortages, the administered price was raised, while if the reverse were true and there were gluts, the administered price was lowered. The obvious question, accepting that administrators really did merely mimic markets was, "Why bother with price administration?" This is a question the Chinese eventually asked themselves, since they subsequently freed most prices to move on their own, a reform the Canadian health care sector has not yet gotten around to.

Three Possible Systems

The most natural way for an economist to think about the health care sector is in terms of "vectors" or lists of prices. Suppose health care involves a thousand different activities. (In fact, it probably involves many more than that.) Imagine each of those activities has a price. Prices can be positive, zero, or, in the case of subsidized goods, negative. The price vector for health care is merely the 1,000-entry list of all the prices charged. Call that list P^M ("M" for medicare). The way medicare is currently run, lots of the entries on the P^M list are zero. But they aren't all zero. Doctors do get paid. Test tubes do get purchased.

Now imagine another list of prices, P^P, which represents the prices for these 1,000 activities that would be produced by a completely private system of health care in which demand and supply operating in open markets ran the system. It's unlikely that many of these prices would be zero, though some might be. If there was a strong social stigma against selling blood or body parts, for instance, allocation of these items might be handled mainly by what has been called "the gift relationship." Or, since someone will always defy prevailing stigma, dual markets might emerge, with some people selling these things and others exchanging them without the intervention of commerce.

Finally, imagine a list of prices P*, the "optimal" list of prices, sometimes referred to as the list of "shadow prices," in which every one of the 1,000 prices is at the "right" level. The obvious question is how to define "right." In economics, the right price is that which produces just the right amount of the activity in question, and the right amount of the activity is where the usefulness (or "utility") of having just a little bit more of it is equal to the usefulness (or "utility") that must be given up in order to produce that little bit more. Why does usefulness have to be given up to produce an activity? Because the effort and resources that go into it could have gone into other useful activities. That may sound circular, but in fact this way of thinking provides a (very useful!) way of comparing the benefits that different activities provide "at the margin"; that is, if they were expanded ever so slightly.

Note that in general, the right price won't be zero (as it is under the kind of first-dollar comprehensive coverage that medicare claims to provide). If it is zero, consumers will have every incentive to keep consuming until they get no use at all from the last unit consumed. But that's justified only if the resources consumed can produce no benefit anywhere else in the society, which seems unlikely in real-world societies. Thus, even in the optimal world, people might have to wait for at least some kinds of surgeries; eliminating all waiting time may simply be too costly, given what has to be sacrificed in other areas by spending enough to keep all the surgeons and operating rooms that might ever be necessary on 24/7 call.

The big question is obviously this: How does P* (the vector of optimal prices), compare with P^P (the prices private markets would produce), and P^M (the prices implicitly or explicitly charged under medicare)? P* is the perfect vector, but the perfect is often the enemy of the good. No real-world system is likely to duplicate P*. But the goal of policy should be to get as close to P* as possible. We have medicare, presumably, because we think it takes us closer to the ideal than private health care would. The fact that medicare is increasingly under challenge means more and more Canadians think that this fact is not true as it once may have been. Let's examine the two systems' failings.

How far away is P^P from P*? There is the obvious problem that, given the existing distribution of income, health care prices — like all prices — will reflect the tastes of the wealthy. Fans of the free market, such as myself, often compare it with a never-ending referendum. People vote with their dollars and they never stop voting. They vote around the clock, all through the calendar. The market responds, not quite instantaneously but usually close enough, to their slightest commercial whim. But this never-ending referendum isn't one person, one vote. The people with the most dollars have the most say about what gets produced. And even if the system does manage to get prices more or less right, non-zero prices will exclude anyone who doesn't have enough money.

The solution to exclusion, however, is to redistribute the dollars. If poor people don't have enough say in the outcome, or can't afford to pay the right price, that situation can be remedied by giving them money. If there are too many electronic scans for rich people's tennis elbows and too few for poor kids' possible brain tumours, put purchasing power in the hands of poor kids' parents and the market will respond. The rich people's tennis elbows will still get their MRI time, but diagnostics companies will find that it now pays to invest in additional machines to check poor people's problems, too. In a market system, property is heft.

Supporters of medicare would respond that even if incomes were distributed more equally — they would probably say "more fairly," though when income has to be earned there's no reason to suppose equal distribution of it is fair — private markets still wouldn't get health care prices right. They'd reason that health care is too complex a product. Consumers don't know what's good for them and therefore can't make an intelligent trade-off between what care costs and how much it's likely to benefit them.

But modern consumers face this dilemma all the time. This essay is being written on a machine that is very complex, much too complex for me to understand. But I have learned that it produces considerable benefits and have contracted with someone who does understand it to help me when it breaks down or when I don't understand how to get something I want from it. I'm writing the paper from an office in my home, also a big, expensive, complex system that I don't fully understand and that put a large hole in my budget when I bought it, which is why I had it inspected by a professional house inspector before signing the agreement to purchase. The market produces advisors of all kinds to help with important, complex purchases. And even if consumers prefer not to hire human advisors, they can read books or search the Web for information about their prospective purchase. More and more of us are highly educated, after all. Buying health care may not be as simple as buying Kraft Dinner, but it is by no means uniquely complex. These days, more and more purchases, from cars to computers to kids' educations, are big, important, and baffling. And, of course, not all health care is mysterious. A broken arm is a broken arm. You know you've broken it and it's more or less obvious what will be involved in fixing it.

So the market's failings may not be disqualifying, but they *are* failings. Poor people may well be frozen out. Reducing their pain and anxiety, if they could afford the right care, might be very "useful," but someone else with better insurance or a greater net worth gets the care instead, even if their problem is not nearly so serious. And patients do sometimes find themselves in a position where they have no idea if what the doctor orders makes any sense at all.

But publicly provided health care isn't perfect, either. By moving the finance of medicare into the public sphere, we in effect require society at large, through the normal processes of representative democracy — that is, politics and bureaucracy — to make the trade-off between finance and care, cost and benefit. We don't provide any and all care that people may demand. We provide the care that our willingness to pay taxes or go without other public services makes possible. The difference between what we would like to have and what our willingness to pay taxes allows us to have is taken up by rationing: people have to wait for services (which favours those, like professors and the unemployed, whose schedules are flexible). Or people go without the services we decide not to cover. Or (the poor excepted) they go to the United States to get them.

Decisions about how much to provide of each of the myriad services medicare involves are inevitably political (which doesn't necessarily mean cynical or expedient, though it doesn't necessarily not mean those things, either). A public official weighs costs and benefits, is petitioned by citizens and interest groups, and makes a decision about which services get how much funding. The goal should be to approximate the shadow price; that is, to provide the amount of each service where the utility gained is just equal to the utility lost in what has to be given up elsewhere. Unfortunately, there are at least four reasons to fear this does not happen:

- Assessing the value of reduced pain or anxiety is obviously difficult.
- The overall amount of money available to the system is determined, not by citizens' feelings about extra health care (as it would be if they were buying it for themselves), but by their willingness to pay taxes and by competing ministers' skill in lobbying for funds for their departments.

- Suppliers will organize and apply pressure in ways that would be unlikely or even impossible if decisions about compensation were genuinely decentralized.
- Prejudice and fad will also enter into the process.

In fact, the degree to which fad runs the system is alarming. In the early 1990s, official Canadian wisdom had it that there were too many doctors, so most jurisdictions encouraged early retirements and reduced medical school spaces, with the result that in the early 2000s, doctors are in short supply. In the mid-1990s, everyone favoured home care, which was used as a justification for cutting back acute care facilities, though usually without a commensurate increase in home care budgets. Now the medicare establishment is infatuated with capitation, salaries, and group practice. Capitation, which gives a doctor a fixed remuneration per patient regardless of how often the patient visits, does address the danger that doctors will "spin" patients in order to increase the fees they receive, but it introduces the new danger that doctors are compensated whether or not they see patients. The theory is that patients can discipline doctors by changing practices, but most capitation schemes put limits on patients' mobility so as to prevent the system from falling into complete confusion. (When, five years or a decade from now, capitation declines in favour, will the return to fee-for-service be known as "decapitation"?)

Putting physicians on salaries creates an even stronger disincentive to see patients: doctors are paid the same no matter how many or few people they treat. The obvious remedy is to require them to see a certain quota of patients per day. How long will it be, however, before the floor becomes a ceiling and a labour union mentality comes to dominate doctor-patient relations? If it's four o'clock, it's time to close, whatever Hippocrates might have said.

There are similar pitfalls in the forced amalgamation of individual practices into round-the-clock clinics, another health policy fad of the early twenty-first century. This may make sense in some circumstances, but it may not in others. If all doctors are centralized in group practices, that may increase the average time patients spend getting to them. No doubt it is convenient to have twenty-four-hour service seven days a week, but the sum of patient inconvenience may actually be greater with centralized services. It is good of the country's ministers of health to point out the possible advantages of group practices, but doctors presumably are capable of figuring these out for themselves. And so long as they continue to be paid on a fee-for-service basis, they can be counted on to introduce innovations that will increase the desire of patients to use their services. Why they should be forced into group practices is not at all clear.

Health ministers, of all ministers, should be wary of the dangers of monoculture. And yet the country swings from one purported panacea to another on roughly a five-year cycle. The Soviet Union has already been mentioned. In the 1940s and 1950s, Stalin's chief geneticist, Trofim Denisovich Lysenko, instituted crackpot ideas designed to increase Soviet agricultural production. Lysenko rejected Mendelian biology and believed that, placed in the appropriate environment, wheat seeds could grow rye. He obviously was not the only problem with Stalinist agriculture, but it should not be surprising that in the years following his tenure as "dictator of biology," crop shortages eventually caused the Soviets to depend on Saskatchewan for their wheat. If Lysenko had merely been the head of an agricultural corporation in a free market agricultural industry, his ideas would have caused disaster for his company and its shareholders and he would have been turfed, with minimal damage to the system at large. But from 1940 to 1965, he was director of the Institute of Genetics at the Academy of Sciences in the U.S.S.R. and as a result, his follies were inflicted on the entire nation.

Canada's current crop of health ministers is not composed of crackpots. Most try to secure the best advice possible before making decisions, and they have taken great strides in recent years to collect useful information about the system they administer. But the decisions they make are, like Lysenko's, system-wide decisions and the cost when these decisions are wrong is borne by us all. In that respect, Canada's health ministers can be every bit as dangerous as Lysenko.

Will More Money Help?

If many of the proffered panaceas for the system cycle in and out, one that does not is the recommendation that more money is needed. Though the system is always said to be short of money, critics of medicare seldom fail to point out that the dollar value of spending has continued to grow, even in some cases on a per capita basis, so the growth of budgets has not prevented the system's current problems.

On the other hand, the critics sometimes fail to control for increases in the cost of health services, so perhaps the rise in spending has not been as sharp as they claim. But if new real-dollar spending was made available, would that solve the problem? An economist cannot help but think that if your problem is shortages, money very likely will help. If you need ten more radiologists and radiologists cost X dollars per year, then a budget increase of ten times X can obviously help. But the money really does have to go to the radiologists, not to some interesting new initiative that catches the eye of the minister or the minister's many deputies. And a shortage of radiologists really does have to be the problem. It can't be that you think radiologists are the problem because they're such good lobbyists, and your problems are really elsewhere.

How much money would be enough? Medicare deals in truly massive amounts of money. Consider the increase in funding that preceded the 2000 federal election. The federal government granted the provinces an extra $23.4 billion for health care, a number that was invoked several times daily during the election campaign and which, in fairness, does sound like a lot. But it isn't really. In the first place, it was actually $21.2 billion, since $2.2 billion was for early childhood education. And it was $21.2 billion over five years, which averages out to $4.24 billion a year. To put things in perspective, in 1999, the last year for which complete data are available, Canadian governments spent a total of $404 billion. So at $4.24 billion, the increase in health care spending that supposedly has saved medicare is just a little over 1 percent of overall public expenditure. Look at it another way: dividing $4.24 billion by the slightly more than 30 million Canadians who are potential users of the system gives an annual increase of just less than $140 per capita on health care spending. The Canadian Institute for Health Information puts current per capita spending on health at about $2,800 a year. So that's just over a 5 percent increase in spending on health care, not counting population (or at least medicare card) growth, assuming the provinces decide to spend the new money on health care.

Some of the money does look like it's pretty well ear-marked: there's $1 billion for a new Medical Equipment Fund. Ottawa has apparently come round to the view that MRI machines and such aren't just self-indulgent American luxuries, but are in fact legitimate tools for diagnosis. With $1 billion to play with, perhaps now Canada will have more MRI machines than, say, Rhode Island.

There's another $500 million for Health Information Technology (which means putting health data onto smart cards), and another $800 million to promote full-service, twenty-four-hour, seven-days-a-week clinics. But the rest of the money isn't ear-marked, and even if the provinces do spend it on health care — an obligation the federal government would have trouble enforcing — it's not clear that it will all get turned into extra care. Some of it will go to increased administration and some to higher costs (i.e., wages) for existing services. That's not necessarily bad — we want our doctors and nurses to stop moving south, and to that end higher salaries clearly help. But just how much of the 5 percent per capita increase does that leave for genuinely new service? Probably not much. The language of the first ministers' document that accompanied the new money suggests they realize this fact. It promised only to provide Canadians with "reasonably timely" access to health care. Canadians don't want "reasonably timely" access. They want timely access, period.

What's to be Done?

If you believe that markets generally allocate resources well, and that the strain medicare currently is under will only increase as the population both ages and becomes ever more resistant to tax increases, you're led to believe that the status quo is not sustainable. That's no great revelation, of course. Virtually every commentary ever written on medicare has said the status quo is unsustainable, even those that then go on to recommend sustaining it (which is a great majority).

One disadvantage of favouring decentralized, market-style solutions to the problems of the health care system is that you can't provide the detailed list of recommendations that make most commentators on health matters sound so crisply authoritative: "Expand service A, cut back on service B, move more into this, withdraw partly from that. That's what we need. Problem solved. Next problem?" By contrast, the essence of decentralization is that no one knows in advance which services and techniques will be adopted. When services are wanted or prove successful, they will grow; when they are not wanted or aren't successful, they won't.

Some general outlines of reform are discernible, however. A first precept for health care policy is that people, especially children, should not be excluded from necessary care simply because they are poor. It is probably inevitable, no matter what system we have, that the rich and influential will get better care than the poor. (In the 1990s, a study of U.S. Medicare — the free health care plan for seniors — found that race and income were significantly correlated with whether people made more intensive use of the system. Poor people and non-whites received less care, even though no one faced user charges.) But, as I concluded sitting in the waiting room of The Vic waiting for my wife's ultrasound, not providing adequate care for people simply because they are poor is a serious indictment of a rich society. Making sure the poor are not excluded can mean giving them enough money to purchase adequate insurance, buying care on their behalf, or allowing them access at forfeitable prices to a system in which most other people pay substantial coinsurance. True, special arrangements for the poor rather than perfectly equal treatment for all may well be stigmatizing. If it is thought desirable to reduce this stigma, computerized administration should make the establishment of different pricing structures virtually anonymous. Who need know that the machines have read a different price off your medicare card than mine? But if stigma cannot be entirely eliminated, a system under increasing stress may simply have to tolerate stigma.

Beyond that, what do you do? The solution favoured by many would-be reformers is some variant or other of medical savings accounts, in which people are given a fixed amount of money each year and are then left free to manage their own health care budget in a system where point-of-contact charging for services becomes the norm.[2] State-provided or -subsidized insurance remains in place to cover so-called catastrophic illness or accident, the kind that can wipe out a family's savings. Relatively small-scale experiments with such a system, including that by at least one small country, Singapore, have proved encouraging.

Singapore is not Canada, however, and Canadians are not usually given to revolutionary change, which is what a wholesale, countrywide switchover to medical savings accounts would be. That does not mean experiments aren't possible, whether on a provincewide basis — could Saskatchewan show the way again? — or within regions of the larger provinces, especially if the federal government were to allow an exception to the Canada Health Act for the purposes of experimentation. But even if this happened, nationwide adoption of medical savings accounts seems a long way off.

In the meantime, change likely will continue on the margins of the system, as Canadians become more and more used to paying for some medical services (especially diagnostics) either out-of-pocket or with private insurance. The system's trajectory is not hard to foretell. As client populations grow and costs rise, the range of core services provided free will decline and more and more items will be accompanied by a charge.

Over time, the supply of fringe services will grow in response to cash-backed patient demand.

How the core evolves will depend on what happens to tax revenues, patient demands, and cost structures within it. If tax revenues remain at current levels and demand pressures on the core ease as the fringe expands, quality of service in the core may stabilize or even improve.

It is often assumed that as the self-financed fringe expands, those relatively well-to-do taxpayers who use it most will resist having to pay twice for health care, first by direct billing and then again in the form of taxes. That may well be their reaction, but whether they can make their desires reality remains to be seen. Much has been made of the "tax revolt" of the 1990s, but as of this writing, in the latest year for which consistent Organisation for Economic Co-Operation and Development data are available, tax revenues were running at an all-time high as a percentage of Canadian GDP — despite the combined influence of Mike Harris, Ralph Klein, and Paul Martin. So even if upper-income Canadians did want to push the system in a given direction, they may continue to be outvoted and the core might therefore continue to be adequately funded. There is also the possibility that many high-income taxpayers would be less angry at the system and less inclined to withdraw funds from it if it no longer stood in the way of their getting the standard of treatment they want for themselves and their families. They may not volunteer extra taxes, but so long as economic growth continues at a satisfactory pace, they may not insist on dramatic reductions in tax rates. Revenues may therefore remain where they are or even rise as the economy grows.

These days the fashion in social science is to talk in terms of "tipping points." It may be that as the system privatizes itself by stealth, just such a tipping point occurs and Canadians and their governments finally become willing to endorse change and formalize it with the introduction of things like medical savings accounts and distinctive payment or pricing arrangements for their poorer co-citizens. The formal acceptance of payment for service and different levels of care for differently endowed Canadians (which we already have in practice) would be ideologically devastating for Canadians who had grown up with the all-for-one, one-for-all ideal of medicare. But it need not be bad for Canadians' health care, nor for the health care system itself. Neither fully private nor free-for-all health care achieves the ideal balance of utility and disutility that economists describe.

But as waiting lines lengthen, populations age, providers' unions grow stronger and more aggressive, and health care technology continues to be reinvented, we may be reaching the point where Canadian public opinion comes to accept that a private system with guarantees for the poor is less imperfect than a public system providing nominally equal, but slow and mediocre care.

NOTES

1. For a discussion of the uninsured in the United States, see David Henderson's essay in this volume.
2. For more on medical savings accounts, see the essays by Fred McMahon and Martin Zelder and David Gratzer in this volume.

HEALTH REFORM ABROAD

Carl Irvine, Johan Hjertqvist, and David Gratzer

"It's an Americanization!" So goes the common response to any suggestion of market-based reforms for health care. Of course, Canada's health care system is unique — no other nation has a Canada Health Act or a Tommy Douglas — but many of the problems our policy-makers struggle with are the same as those facing health administrators elsewhere. By adopting this knee-jerk attitude, Canadians have deprived themselves of the opportunity to learn from experimentation in other countries. In this essay, economist Carl Irvine and Swedish health expert Johan Hjertqvist join me to discuss market-based reforms in other developed countries.

Public-private partnerships, user fees, and private insurance are taboo topics in Canada. But as we observe, "Many developed countries, often countries with strong socialist backgrounds, have adopted a myriad of market or quasi-market mechanisms to try and enhance the quality of their health care systems. Moreover, they have often achieved impressive results."

This essay opens with a lengthy consideration of the Swedish experience. While this Nordic country is a bastion of government activity and regulation, Stockholm has become a hotbed of public-private partnerships. Among the health services privatized in recent years: home care, laboratory work, ambulance service, and long-term care. A major hospital was recently sold to a private company. Though controversial, the Swedish enthusiasm for privatization has a very simple motivation: it saves money. Lab costs, for instance, fell by 50 percent after being contracted out.

Britain's National Health Service (NHS) was once a model for Canadian health care. Indeed, the NHS was the model Canadians used when contemplating a national health insurance. If our historic roots are tied to the United Kingdom, Canadian reluctance to consider market-based reforms is not. In the NHS, internal market mechanisms were created under a Conservative government, but expanded under a Labour one. Experiments with market-based reforms have also included a significant contracting out of services. The recently reelected Blair government, for instance, pledged during the election campaign to privatize 200,000 surgeries over the next four years.

This essay surveys health reform in a variety of countries. It finds that "many developed countries have some sort of cost-sharing mechanism (such as user fees) to encourage appropriate use of health care services. All these countries have what Canadians would call a 'two-tier' health care system, in that they allow people to seek medical treatment outside the public system. And . . . many countries are moving toward increased competition in the provision of health care through the contracting out of services to the private sector."

While it's difficult to generalize an individual nation's experiences, what emerges from this review is a better understanding of the extent to which countries are embracing market-based reforms. Some experiments are clearly more successful than others. Still, international experience makes a powerful argument for Canadians to begin thinking outside the box.

1. Introduction

"Let the market take over health care!"
—Eva Fernvall, Chair, Swedish National Union of Nurses

In Canada, health care falls under provincial control. In many ways, discussion about health reform has become provincial — not in the jurisdictional sense of the word, but metaphorically. Instead of drawing from the experiences of other nations, Canadians tend to look internally.

There is nothing wrong with learning from our own successes and failures. One of the advantages of Canadian federalism for health care (federal funding but provincial administration) is that we have the potential for ten major laboratories of experimentation. Still, our health care discussions tend to be too insular. And when we do look abroad, the tendency is merely to gaze south.

Unquestionably, Canada's health care system is unique. No other nation has a Canada Health Act or a Tommy Douglas. Indeed, every health care system in the Western world has its own variations in organization. That isn't surprising. Health care systems across the West are influenced by many different (and often local) forces: history, customs, and legislative frameworks. But just as any nation's exact approach to health care may be unique, there are great similarities among Western countries in their aims. Politicians campaign in Berlin on a promise of quality health care, just as they do in Brandon or Barrie.

And there are great similarities in the problems faced by all Western health care systems. Aging demographics and the consequences of the "high-tech, high-expense" medical revolution will not only impact the ability of the Ontario government to deliver timely and effective cancer care, it will influence the Greater Council of Stockholm's ability to do the same for its citizens. And public angst about health care and health reforms isn't just a Canadian phenomenon. In the pubs of London, ON, citizens discuss issues of quality and access just as people do in the pubs of London, England.

Reforming health care along the lines of individual choice and competition — what some would loosely call market-based reforms — is often attacked in Canada as an "Americanization." As noted by David Henderson in his essay in this volume, Canadians have a skewed view of U.S. medicine. More importantly, by dismissing all market reforms, we are deprived of the opportunity to study (and learn from) other countries' experiences.

Public-private partnerships, user fees, private insurance. These topics are taboo in Canada. Many developed countries, often countries with strong socialist backgrounds, have adopted a myriad of market or quasi-market mechanisms to try and enhance the quality of their health care systems. Moreover, they have often achieved impressive results.

This essay opens with a quotation endorsing private medicine. Eva Fernvall isn't a libertarian economist or a profit-minded entrepreneur; she is chair of Sweden's nurses' union. For a variety of reasons, traditional supporters of government involvement in health care (like Fernvall, Labour politicians in Britain, and social democrats in the Netherlands), have come to see that there is an important place for market-based reforms.

This essay will look at the role of markets-based reforms in several developed countries, with particular emphasis on Sweden and the United Kingdom.[1] We show that many nations are considering (or have implemented) many reforms of this type. Indeed, Canadian reluctance is exceptional, bucking an international trend toward more individual choice and competition in health care. More importantly, in many developed countries with health care systems not unlike our own, market mechanisms not only play a greater role in the health care system, but they often help achieve cost savings and reduce waiting times for care.

2. The Swedish Experience

Sweden offers its citizens a cradle-to-grave welfare state, devoted to achieving social equity. To this end, Sweden allocates an astonishing 60 percent of its GDP to government spending.[2] Thus, it would seem counterintuitive to begin with Sweden when considering market-based reforms. Yet in this Nordic bastion of social democracy, the last decade has seen surprising and aggressive experimentation with market reforms.

Sweden's 1990s health reforms are particularly interesting from a Canadian perspective because they were motivated by many of the same problems that have plagued Canada's medicare. Between 1960 and 1980, Sweden's health care spending spiralled upward.[3] As seen in Canada in the early 1990s, Swedish governments in the 1980s sought to control rapidly escalating costs (a problem exacerbated by deficit spending and tax fatigue) and growing public dissatisfaction.

If the reasons for reform are familiar to a Canadian, the result of budgetary restraint is as well: health spending slowed in the late 1980s in Sweden, but with unsatisfactory results. Swedes found their beloved health care system marred by problems: diminished access to primary care, long waiting lists, and difficulty in attracting and retaining staff (particularly nurses and doctors).[4]

Faced with increasingly disenchanted voters, the Swedish government decided that "radical" changes had to be considered. In 1992, the National Care Guarantee was passed.

The goal was clear: Reduce waiting times for patients. The Guarantee was literally a guarantee — patients who waited too long for certain procedures would be issued a voucher and freed to go anywhere in the country for the care they needed.

To the casual observer, this relatively simple reform had an immediate impact: between 1992 and the end of 1993, waiting times shrunk by 22 percent.[5] But the impact of this document was probably limited; there was no financial penalty for lengthy waiting lists, nor did every jurisdiction actually implement the voucher system. If the National Care Guarantee was bold, it was probably more symbolic than substantive. By 1995, waiting lists were again long and growing.[6]

But the National Care Guarantee marked a formal recognition of a problem: waiting lists. Around this same time, the government put in place two reforms in health financing.

The first major change was in hospital funding. Before 1992, hospitals were given block funding (a global budget) regardless of use. After the reforms, patients could pick and choose the hospital that provided them with elective care instead of being assigned to a facility based on geography. Hospitals were also provided with incentives to meet standards.

The intent of this reform was to promote competition among public hospitals. Hospitals now had an incentive to improve their quality and efficiency to attract more patients. Since hospitals could not compete with prices, they could only attract more patients by improving services or reducing waiting times.

By changing the financing system and promoting patient choice, hospital care was transformed. If hospitals were now freer to innovate, they also had good cause: funding was no longer a certainty — it followed the patient. Hospitals began working to seek out new efficiencies and to attract and satisfy patients. They also worked to increase transparency: waiting times for basic procedures at Swedish hospitals are posted on the Internet.

The second major reform was the introduction of an internal market for health care. Modelled after reforms in Britain and New Zealand, health funding was devolved to twenty-six county and city councils. Councils, then, were charged with "buying" services on behalf of their constituents.

Under the old system, medical services were both provided and paid for by the council in each of Sweden's twenty-six districts. Hospitals were managed directly by the councils. Under the new reforms, as in the United Kingdom, a separate public purchaser (the council) was established, and hospitals and other health care providers had to compete for public funds. And, like in the United Kingdom, the response was mixed. Initially, only six counties actually attempted to purchase services. The purchaser-provider split existed only on paper in many parts of Sweden.[7]

If some councils hesitated, some plunged ahead with innovative initiatives. The Greater Council of Stockholm in particular became a hotbed for public-private partnerships. Faced with stagnant public sector monopolies, the Stockholm government sought to improve performance by increasing competition. In 1993 and in 1994, the Stockholm council licensed private providers. Costs plummeted. Public-private partnerships (public financing with private provision) included home care, ambulance services, and laboratory and diagnostic testing.

In less than two years, laboratory costs fell by 50 percent. Monies were also saved elsewhere: support staff services dropped by 30 percent; ambulance costs, by 15 percent.[8] By the time the centre-right government in Stockholm lost the election in 1994, 150 small- and medium-sized contractors had been established to provide health care services.[9]

Moreover, these reforms were so successful that the Socialist government that came to power in 1994 did nothing to reverse them, although they slowed the private providers' rate of growth. All but one of the original private providers survived.[10] With the return to office of the centre-right coalition in 1998, the pace of reform picked up once again. Since that year, 150 health care units have started the process of becoming private companies within the public health care system.

The largest such company, Praktikertjänst, is a producer cooperative, owned by the doctors, nurses, and support staff. The cooperative's 2,300 practices have been able to offer its patients and workers all the benefits of a small, decentralized operation, while controlling administrative costs.[11] Many small and medium producers are joining, or have joined, this cooperative.

Emboldened by their successes, the Greater Council of Stockholm looked for new services to privatize. In 1999, St. George's Hospital, one of Stockholm's largest, was sold to Capio Ltd., a private company. In its first year, it realized savings 10 to 15 percent higher than those achieved by the best-run public hospital, and savings of 15 to 20 percent over the average of the publicly run hospitals.[12]

What is more, it seems the Stockholm government is intent on continuing this process. Of the remaining seven publicly owned hospitals in Stockholm, two have been turned into commercially viable (hence saleable) council-owned companies; two more became council companies in 2001. The remaining three are "candidates" for marketization.[13] It is possible that all of Stockholm's hospitals may be sold, although the hospital companies are being required to prove their efficiency before any decisions are made.

Nursing homes have experienced similar savings where privately contracted public homes have costs that are 20 to 30 percent lower than their public equivalents.[14] Even among medical specialists, Stockholm has seen increased efficiency as a result of contracting out. While public specialists spend more time bogged down with paper work, private specialists have started focusing on spending time with patients. As a result, their budget requests are 10 to 15 percent lower than those of their public colleagues.[15]

With so much success, it's not surprising that the public-private experimentation continues. Right now, there are over 100 health care units leaving public ownership to form private companies. These new contractors include medical and surgical clinics, GP (general practitioner) group practices, laboratories, and psychiatric out-of-hospital clinics. After completion of the latest round of privatizations, some 80 percent of Stockholm's primary care and 40 percent of total health services will be contracted out.

If public-private partnerships have proven popular with health administrators eager to find cost savings and patients hoping for prompt care, there is another group delighted with the experimentation: providers.

Many of the new contractors are nurses keen to increase their salaries and decrease the frustration of working under a bureaucracy.[16] The chair of the Swedish National Union of Nurses, Eva Fernvall, made headlines in 1997 when she said, "Let the market take over health care!"[17] She went on to say that, "in today's society, the old [health care] model no longer works . . . now there is a need for flexibility, entrepreneurship and new channels to let loose the complexity of demand and supply, held back for decades when it comes to health care services. . . . More independent organizations . . . can offer very large gains for Swedish welfare — a better function of welfare at the same or lower cost."[18]

For nurses, privatization has led to increased flexibility and entrepreneurship, but it has also led to higher wages and better working conditions, as nurses wages have increased far faster since the introduction of market reforms than they did prior to them.[19]

Furthermore, despite the fears of critics, the decline in overall health care quality that had been predicted at the beginning of the reforms never materialized. Waiting lists in Stockholm have fallen by two-thirds since the introduction of market reforms; they are a fraction of those in counties that have not embraced the private sector.[20] Even compared with counties that have tepidly innovated, Stockholm has done well. Consider national statistics. Heart surgery patients wait 2 weeks in Stockholm, but 15 to 25 weeks elsewhere in the country, and hip replacement candidates wait 3 to 10 weeks in Stockholm, as opposed to 45 to 50 weeks outside of the capital.[21] For ordinary prostate surgery, a patient typically waits 4 weeks in Stockholm and between 90 and 156 weeks in most parts of Sweden.[22]

In short, market-oriented health reforms in Sweden have been successful. They have controlled costs and boosted health care productivity, while at the same time bettering working conditions for health care providers. More importantly, they sharply reduced waiting times for patients.

The biggest change in Sweden, however, has been a change in mentality, which has moved away from tolerance of problems to a desire to make care patient-focused and competitive.[23] As coauthor Johan Hjertqvist observes, "This 'reform of perceptions' is even more important than changes in techniques and formal incentives."

3. Market Mechanisms in Britain

Historically, British experimentation with public health care was of major interest in Canada. The establishment of the British National Health Service (NHS) in 1948 — with a promise of free and unlimited provisions of medical services and the nationalization of most of the country's medical facilities — popularized the idea of public health care in this country.

As in Canada, initial public enthusiasm waned over the decades. As costs soared, the British government started rationing health care; waiting lists grew while patient satisfaction decreased.

If these problems sound familiar, they are. And if the NHS once served as an inspiration for health reform in this country in the 1950s and 1960s, its reforms in the last decade may also prove of value. Many of these reforms are market-based, either in the form of internal markets or public-private partnerships.

The first of these reforms, started in 1991, was intended to create a market-like system within the context of a publicly funded and publicly operated health care system. This "internal market" introduced a split between health care purchasers and health care providers. The purchasers were the regional health authorities who were given responsibility for funding health care for a population geographically defined by the central government. GPs could also become "fundholders," if they wished. This option provided them with a budget to purchase some services (notably elective surgeries) for their patients. Institutional providers (hospitals) became self-governing trusts within the public sector.

The idea behind these reforms was simple: providers would have to compete with one another to win contracts from the purchasers, be they health authorities or fundholders. Hospitals and service providers would reduce waiting lists and improve the quality of care to win new contracts. The hope was that these new reforms would provide both providers and purchasers alike with incentives to improve performance.

The results of the internal market reforms have been mixed. Health care productivity rose after the 1991 reforms. Whereas productivity increased at 1.5 percent per year over the 1980s, it grew at 2 percent per year in the first half of the 1990s.[24] On the other hand, overall administrative costs rose.[25]

In large part, the internal market reform was not so successful because it retained many of the features of the old NHS. Health authorities could not keep or invest any surplus funds at the end of the year, so they had little incentive to be frugal. Hospitals had little ability to innovate given that surplus monies reverted to the NHS.

More problematic still was the fact that many hospitals depended on huge grants from local health authorities. In a truly competitive environment, hospitals would compete directly with clinics and smaller institutions for funding. This opened the door to a politically harsh possibility: the bankruptcy and closure of hospitals.

Local authorities, pressured by politicians, would not accept this possibility and continued the old practice of block grants to hospitals.[26] Thus, for hospital-based care, the internal market existed in government documents only. Indeed, the lack of success of the internal market in Britain was largely due, not to the failure of competition, but rather to the lack thereof.

This point is reinforced by the relative success of the GP fundholders. Unlike the health authorities, the GP fundholders could retain their surpluses, allowing them to invest in better computer systems, diagnostic tools, and support staff. Because individually they accounted for relatively small budgets, GP fundholders had great flexibility in contracting with local hospitals. Relative to other family doctors, fundholders restrained costs. More importantly, access to care for their patients was enhanced.[27]

Despite their earlier claims to the contrary, the Blair Labour government has preserved internal markets. Under its new plan, the provider-purchaser split remains, although with an emphasis on cooperation rather than competition. The Labour government is also retaining — and expanding — the role of fundholders. Under Labour, GPs are compelled to join primary care groups, effectively a modified fundholding scheme.[28] Moreover, unlike under the previous reforms, both trusts and primary care groups are allowed to retain any surpluses.

Thus, the Thatcher reforms to Britain's NHS have not been undone by Blair. In fact, the opposite is true: his government has undone some of the earlier design flaws. Blair, one could argue, has better enhanced market mechanisms in the public system than did Margaret Thatcher.[29]

The influence of the market in Britain is not restricted to the public system. Private insurance and privately funded health care play a complementary role to the NHS. Indeed, in 1997, private insurance companies, friendly societies, and a range of Health Cash Benefit Schemes covered over 12 million people for medical expenses.[30] There are 210 private hospitals with 11,000 beds in Britain, and over 600 operating theaters.[31] In addition, the independent sector — as the British call for-profit and not-for-profit providers outside of the NHS — provides 20 percent of all acute elective surgeries, and 30 percent of all hip replacements.

Nor does the independent sector just perform relatively simple surgeries; it provides one million procedures every year and almost one-quarter of these are classified as major or major/complex surgeries, such as heart bypasses.[32] And, according to Dr. Tim Evans, the executive director of public affairs at the Independent Healthcare Association, the independent sector accounts for 15,000 nursing homes, with 420,000 beds.[33]

The NHS also relies on private services. Public-private partnerships cover a variety of areas. Baxter Healthcare, a private company, runs most of the dialysis in Britain. Pathology labs, too, are contracted out. And locally, many communities are looking to private providers. The county council of Berkshire just signed a contract with a company to operate the majority of residential homes in the district.

Almost 75 percent of the patients housed in these private nursing homes are financed, either in full or in part, by the public sector.[34] The role of the independent sector in home care is also increasing. Although it remains largely funded by the public sector — mostly local governments — the percentage of home care provided by the independent sector has been steadily increasing, and now accounts for over 50 percent of home care services provided.[35] Furthermore, almost 90 percent of acute brain injury rehabilitation in Britain is done by the independent sector.[36]

Much of this change has occurred under Prime Minister Tony Blair's Labour government. Are the Blairites dismayed by the increased role of private medicine within the public system? Actually, the opposite is true. The Independent Healthcare Association — the umbrella group for private providers in Great Britain — recently signed a Concordat with Tony Blair's government. The *Financial Times* called the Concordat one of the most important documents in the fifty-year history of the National Health Service. Titled *For the Benefit of Patients*, it enables NHS-funded patients who need intensive care or elective surgery to receive such services in independent sector hospitals.

The agreement begins with the historic words "there should be no organisational or ideological barriers to the delivery of high quality healthcare free at the point of delivery to those who need it."[37] It goes on to announce a "commitment towards planning the use of private and voluntary health care providers, not only at times of pressure but also on a more proactive longer term basis where this offers demonstrable value for money and high standards for patients."

Why is a Labour government keen on public-private partnerships? For one thing, it makes fiscal sense. The Adam Smith Institute estimates that contracting out reduces costs by about 20 percent.

Not surprisingly, then, even prior to the Concordat, the NHS was contracting with private hospitals. According to Dr. Evans, almost 100,000 surgeries were provided to NHS patients by the private sector between 1997 and 2000.[38] The Concordat is expected to increase the number of privately provided and publicly funded operations substantially. Although it is still early, the initial response seems positive.[39]

The Labour Party embraces the private sector as a partner in the NHS. Its 2001 election manifesto promised to "work with the private sector to use spare capacity . . . for NHS patients."[40] Part of the pledge includes the promise of new surgical centres to be run and managed by the private sector. The centres will relieve NHS operating theatres of 200,000 procedures by 2004.

The Institute for Public Policy Research was calling for a much larger role for the private sector. The Blairite think tank — asked to study these issues by the Prime Minister himself — advocates private sector involvement in everything from the administrative services for family doctors' offices to the contracting out of cardiac and neurosurgeries. The report even flirts with the idea of a privately run and managed hospital. Though the Labour platform didn't endorse these ideas, it didn't rule them out, either.

It seems that British policy-makers, especially the Labourites, have overcome concerns about private health providers. No wonder. The evidence suggests that market mechanisms can be successful at enhancing the quality of health care received, while reducing costs.

4. Market Reforms in Other Nations

While the United Kingdom and Sweden offer strong examples of market-based health reforms, the British and Swedish experiences are not isolated. Even a cursory glance at the health systems of other developed countries shows a willingness and interest to attempt reforms that would be unthinkable in Canada.

The following table provides a summary of market-based reforms used in various countries, mostly European.

TABLE 1

Market Mechanisms in Selected Countries

Country	User Fees[1]			Contracting out of services to private sector	Purchaser-provider split in public system	Private health insurers within public system[2]	Private health care complementary to public system[3]
	GP	Specialist	Hospital				
Australia	Yes	Yes	No	Yes	No	NA	Yes
Finland	Yes**	Yes**	Yes	Yes	Yes	NA	Yes
France	Yes*	Yes	Yes	Yes	Yes	NA	Yes
Germany	No	No	Yes**	Yes	Yes	Yes	Yes
Ireland	Yes*	Yes*	Yes*	Yes	No	NA	Yes
Israel	Yes	Yes	Yes	Yes	Yes	Yes	Yes
Italy	No	Yes	Yes	Yes	Yes	NA	Yes
Netherlands	No	Yes**	Yes**	Yes	Yes	Yes	Yes
Norway	Yes**	Yes**	No	Yes	No	NA	Yes
South Africa	Yes*	No	No	Yes	No	NA	Yes
Sweden	Yes*,**	Yes**	Yes	Yes	Yes	NA	Yes
Switzerland	Yes*	Yes*	Yes**	(Yes)	Yes	Yes	Yes
United Kingdom	No	No	No	Yes	Yes	NA	Yes

1. Indicates whether public health care system charges user fees for General Practitioner visits (GP), outpatient specialist visits (Specialist), and inpatient hospital treatment (Hospital). * indicates that the particular user fees is waived for some groups of patients, usually based on income, age, health condition. ** indicates that there is a maximum level of user fees which can be charged in a given period.
2. In countries with social insurance models of health care financing.
3. A private health care system is complementary if one can obtain the same services within the private system as one could in the public system. Canadians would probably call this "two-tier" health care.

Several trends clearly emerge.

First, many developed countries have some sort of cost-sharing mechanism (such as user fees) to encourage appropriate use of health care services. Second, all these countries have what Canadians would call a "two-tier" health care system, in that they allow people to seek medical treatment outside of the public system. And third, many countries are moving toward increased competition in the provision of health care through the contracting out of services to the private sector (as in Finland, Germany, and Sweden).

On the latter point, informal Blair advisor and former Fabian Society Research Director Stephen Pollard observes, "Across . . . Europe the story is the same — politicians of Left and Right treat such cooperation between state and independent providers as normal, making much more money available to serve patients' needs."[41]

Even countries with a traditional social insurance–style health care system are moving toward competition, including private sector contractors, among health care purchasers. Geert Jan Hamilton, the director of legislation at the Dutch Health Ministry, observes, "The whole provider side of [Dutch] health care is basically private. Providers undergo the influence of regulation but they are basically private entities. The insurance side is private as well, but [regulated] under a social security system."[42]

Consider health reforms in the following countries:

Australia

While similar to the Canadian health care system, Australia's allows physicians to extra-bill in the public system.

Australia also allows private insurance. Before recent reforms, private insurance covered almost 6.4 million people.[43] Private hospitals account for 30.4 percent of total admissions, and 25.3 percent of total bed days.[44]

In response to fiscal pressures, the government has encouraged patients to shift to the private sector through

- the use of a variety of tax subsidies for all citizens, and
- modest financial penalties for wealthy citizens who remain in the public system.

Enrollment in private plans now approaches 45 percent of the population.[45]

Finland

As in Sweden and the U.K., Finland has started to move toward a public contract model of health care; that is, a publicly financed system, with a variety of public, not-for-profit, and for-profit providers.[46]

Finland also has a system of user fees, which vary by municipality, but which are, at most, $9 per visit, $18 a year for GP and specialist visits, and $23 per day for hospital inpatient services.[47]

France

User fees are applied to most medical services, but are waived for specific diseases (AIDS, diabetes, etc.) and for special chronic care cases.[48] One-third of French hospitals are private.[49] Doctors are allowed to opt out of the public system and charge supplemental fees.[50]

Germany

Germany has a compulsory social insurance scheme for individuals below a certain income level (accounting for roughly 90 percent of the population) and private health insurers for the remainder of the population if they choose to opt out of the public system.[51]

Within the public Social Insurance Schemes (SIS), the German government has started to embrace the following quasi-market mechanisms to encourage cost savings and improvements in quality of care:

- Increasingly, for-profit health insurance providers compete with public insurances, though insurance providers are not allowed to exclude people based on health status.
- Insurance providers are also encouraged to negotiate prices among hospital associations to reduce costs.
- All insurances have a mandatory user fee of $7 a day (for up to fourteen days) for inpatient hospital care.[52]
- The vast majority of public hospitals are currently being privatized. By 2015, it is expected that only a few hundred of Germany's 1,700 hospitals will remain under the control of the state.[53]

Ireland

Ireland has means-tested user fees, meaning that roughly one-third of the population is exempt while the rest must make copayments. Those in the latter group must make copayments for GP visits: $8 a visit up to $56 a month for specialist services; and for inpatient hospital care in the public ward, they are charged $27 a day up to $270 a year.[54]

Almost 14 percent of Ireland's hospital beds are in private hospitals.[55]

Doctors serve both public and private patients, and indeed many doctors practise in both public and private hospitals.[56] The Irish government does not see private health care as a threat to the public system; rather, it sees it as playing "a complementary role."

Israel

Israel offers health insurance (subscribed to on a voluntary basis) through four not-for-profit sick funds. In the past, switching among sick funds was difficult.

In the mid-1990s, Israel reformed health care with the National Health Insurance Law. Now, sick funds must provide a basic and uniform package of entitlements. Premiums for the sick funds are risk-adjusted. The centre-piece of the reform: citizens can easily switch among sick funds, in effect creating competition.

Patient satisfaction with health care has increased, and the proportion of sick fund members reporting an improvement in quality has increased and waiting times for GPs and specialists have fallen.[57] The professionalism of health care providers and the cleanliness of health care facilities are perceived to have improved with increased competition between health care purchasers.[58]

Netherlands

As in Germany, the Netherlands has traditionally provided health care through a social insurance scheme. Before recent reforms, many problems existed. Sickness funds were fully reimbursed by the government, which provided little incentive for cost containment. Patients had no choice among sickness funds, which reduced the funds' responsiveness to patient needs.

The Netherlands' provision of health care has undergone significant change. Reforms include the following:

- Sickness funds and private insurers compete directly with one another for customers.
- Purchasers must provide a uniform set of entitlements at a flat-rate premium. These funds receive grants from the central government based on the age, sex, region, and disability status of their members.
- Sickness funds are allowed to contract selectively with providers, a move intended to promote competition among providers.
- Sickness funds now have to bear a portion, albeit a small one, of high health care costs, so they have an incentive to restrain costs.

264 ◆ BETTER MEDICINE

Norway

Norway maintains a system of copayments to ensure appropriate utilization of services.

The Norwegian user fee schedule includes a $17 user fee per GP consultation ($23 on evenings or weekends) and a $16 user fee for specialist visits. The user fees are waived once a patient has reached a yearly maximum of $138.[59]

South Africa

Faced with spiralling costs associated with the AIDS crisis, as well as expanded primary care programs, the Nelson Mandela government sought to reduce public expenses by encouraging citizens to opt for private insurance. To this end, South Africa deregulated the insurance market in the mid-1990s. Medical savings account-type plans are currently the most popular option.

Switzerland

Switzerland has universal insurance, but costs are largely borne privately.[60] This is achieved by making health insurance compulsory. Plans are offered both by the public and private sectors. To offset insurance costs, the poor (means-tested) receive grants to purchase insurance. Insurance companies cannot refuse high-risk patients, but government offers special subsidies to offset the higher costs.

Switzerland also has a cost-sharing arrangement with patients to ensure responsible use of services. Everyone has a uniform $100 deductible, plus a $112 deductible for GP and specialist services, plus a 10 percent copayment on all costs. Moreover, citizens must also pay $7 a day for in-patient hospital care.[61]

5. Lessons from Abroad

Sarah Polley, the actor known for her roles in *Guinevere* and *Go*, made headlines when she helped organize a music concert at the University of Toronto. What would drive a star like Polley to leave Cannes for Convocation Hall? Polley wants to fight the privatization of Ontario's health care system.

"We're the kind of society . . . that believes in public health care and public education. Those are the things that define being Canadian and if that changes, I don't know why I'm so militant about staying here."[62] In fact, Polley went further, telling the *Toronto Star* that she feels so strongly, she may move.

Quick question: Where is Polley moving to?

Many Canadian politicians, policy analysts, and celebrities maintain that market-based reforms are just a way of Americanizing medicare. The survey in this essay about health reforms in other countries shows the extent to which developed countries — often ones with rich social democratic roots — are willing to experiment with innovative approaches to health financing and delivery.

Because the health care debate is so emotional, Canadian participants have a tendency to overstate their case. Testifying before a Senate committee, a University of Toronto academic explained her opposition to user fees: New Zealand implemented user fees and suffers from poor infant mortality rates. It doesn't take a Ph.D in health administration to see the flaw in this argument. For one thing, many countries have user fees, some with far better infant mortality rates than Canada's. More importantly, infant mortality rates reflect complex interactions of social and economic conditions, not just access to care. The success or failure of user fees cannot be gleaned by one statistic in a single nation.

Likewise, it would be equally simplistic to make sweeping generalizations about the efficacy of market-based reforms. There is no single solution for Canada's health care woes.

But the above survey does shed some light on the issue. In particular, it serves to rebut many of the arguments put forward today in Canada. *Contracting out increases costs.* Evidence from Britain and Sweden suggests the opposite. *User fees are not used anywhere but in the United States.* Most nations have user fees for basic medical and hospital services. *Private insurance corrupts the public system.* Every Western country (but Canada) allows a private option; some rely on it to reduce strain on the government-backed system, going so far as to offer tax subsidies.

Of course, many of the reforms mentioned in this essay are controversial. And many of the health care systems described here are deeply troubled — even after years of change.

Bear in mind two points. First, international studies like the one recently conducted by the Harvard School of Public Health suggest that, in terms of waiting times and perceived quality, Canada ranks poorly. Second, the Canadian phobia of market-based health reforms is practically unparalleled in the West. If such initiatives are as damaging as critics claim, why do the Brits and Swedes forge ahead? Why isn't a single country listed in this essay considering a Canada Health Act to call its own?

NOTES

1. Hereafter, when we use the term "market" we include the private health care sector, but also include internal markets in the context of a publicly run system, as well as market-type mechanisms such as user fees.
2. Finn Diderichsen, "Sweden," *Journal of Health Politics, Policy, and Law* 25.5 (2000): 931.
3. Ibid.
4. Ibid.
5. Johan Calltorp and Michael Harrison, "The Reorientation of Market-Oriented Reforms in Swedish Health-Care," *Health Policy* 50 (2000): 223.
6. The waiting list figures are drawn from national data on waiting times for twelve specific diagnoses, including bladder stone, cataracts, and operable coronary artery disease. In 1992, 52,000 Swedes waited for care. In 1993, 40,000 were waiting. By 1995, the lists were growing again. What accounted for the short-term drop? Perhaps the answer lies more in the surge in health funding. As in Canada and Great Britain, dramatic increases in spending appear to temporarily address demand problems.
7. Even today, only about half the councils have a purchaser-provider split.
8. Frontier Center for Public Policy, "Conversations from the Frontier, No. 12," 31 Jan. 2001, www.fcpp.org/publications/conversations/hjertqvist.html. (Much of the data from the Stockholm experiment comes directly from the Greater Council of Stockholm. Notes, thus, are meant to provide additional sources of information.)
9. Peter Holle and Michel Kelly-Gagnon, "How Swedish Socialists Chose Private Health Care," *National Post*, 3 Oct. 2000, C19.
10. Ibid.
11. Ibid.
12. Johan Hjertqvist, "The Purchaser-Provider Split: Swedish Health-Care Reform," 20 Feb. 2001, www.fcpp.org/publications/backgrounders/sweden.html.
13. FCPP, "Conversations."
14. Hjertqvist, "The Purchaser-Provider Split."
15. Holle and Kelly-Gagnon, "How Swedish Socialists Chose Private Health Care."
16. FCPP, "Conversations."
17. Ibid.
18. Hjertqvist, "The Purchaser-Provider Split."
19. Ibid.
20. Frontier Center for Public Policy, "Is Profit a Poison Pill for Health Care?" 22 Feb. 2001, www.fcpp.org/publications/policy_notes/spr/health_care/feb232001.pdf.
21. Ibid.

22. For a more extensive comparison of waiting lists in Sweden, see Johan Hjertqvist, "Swedish Healthcare In Transition: The Internet Empowers Swedish Healthcare Consumers," Frontier Centre for Public Policy, May 2001, www.fcpp.org.

23. A good example of the patient-oriented innovation occurring in Stockholm is the present initiative to develop Web portals for every citizen, which will provide personal health information and assistance in making health care–related decisions. Using a communications tool of choice — a personal computer, a cell phone, wireless application protocol (WAP) — a person will be able to subscribe to weekly medical advice, a monthly electronic newsletter, or a symptoms guide. The individual will be able to get updated news on waiting times for the kind of treatment needed. As well, portals will be personalized to address medical conditions. So, for example, if a person suffers from asthma, he or she can build a database of information, including lists of clinics and providers, relevant medication therapies, crisis instructions, forecasts on air pollution, support groups, and research reports.

24. Julian Legrand, "Competition, Cooperation, or Control? Tales from the British National Health Service," *Health Affairs* 10.3 (1999): 30.

25. Ibid., 31.

26. Ibid., 33.

27. Rudolf Klein, "Why Britain is Reorganizing its National Health Service — Yet Again," *Health Affairs* 17.4 (1998): 118.

28. Legrand, "Competition, Cooperation, or Control?" 36.

29. As Stephen Pollard, an informal Blair advisor and a former research director for the Fabian Society, explains, "Replacing the old GP fundholders, who had their own budget, with much larger Primary Care Groups, where groups of GPs come together and spend their own aggregate budgets, has been seized on by some of the more go-ahead practices as providing them with far more negotiating and spending clout than they ever had under the Conservatives reforms." Stephen Pollard, "The Impatient Patient-Lessons From the U.K.," *Reinventing Health Care*, Helen Brown, ed. (London: Social Market Foundation, 2000), 32.

30. Adrian Bull and Yvonne Doyle, "Role of Private Sector in United Kingdom Healthcare System," *British Medical Journal* 321 (2000): 563.

31. Tim Evans, interview with Carl Irvine, London, England, 18 May 2001.

32. Ibid.

33. This translates into a staggering 150 million bed days per year.

34. Evans, interview.

35. Ibid.

36. Ibid.

37. Department of Health, "Introduction," *A Concordat with the Private and Voluntary Health Care Provider Sector*, 31 Oct. 2000, www.doh.gov.uk/commissioning/guidance.htm#concordat.

38. Evans, interview.

39. According to BUPA, a private health insurance provider, the number of public patients treated by their private hospitals increased almost threefold in the three months from October to December 2000 compared with the same months a year earlier. See Jeremy Laurance, "Number of NHS Patients Treated Privately Soars to Boost Private Sector," *The Independent*, 19 Feb. 2000, 6. As well, according to Dr. Evans, in the first quarter of 2001 alone, almost 25,000 publicly funded surgeries took place in the independent sector, almost three times the rate between 1997 and 2000.

40. Labour Party, *Ambitions For Britain: Labour's Manifesto 2001*, 16 May 2000, 7, www. labour.org.uk/Eng1-www.pdf.
41. Stephen Pollard, "The Case For Private Mutual Health Care: A Socialist View," *Pfizer Forum*, 1995, www.pfizerforum.com/english/pollard.shtml.
42. Geert Jan Hamilton, "Innovations in Dutch Health Care," in *Reinventing Health Care*, 1.
43. Christopher Zinn, "Australia Moves to Boost Private Health Cover," *British Medical Journal* 321 (2000): 10.
44. Jane Hall, "Incremental Change in the Australian Health Care System," *Health Affairs* 18.3 (1999): 98.
45. Greg Scandlen, "Australia Ends Community Rating," *NCPA's Health Policy Week No. 169*, 3 June 2001. Based on Sharon Willcox, "Promoting Private Health Insurance In Australia," *Market Watch, Health Affairs*, May/June 2001.
46. Wynand van de Ven, "Market-Oriented Health Care Reforms: Trends and Future Options," *Social Science & Medicine* 43.5 (1996): 656.
47. Diana Delnoij, Peter Groenewegen, and Corina Ros, "All Rights Reserved, or Can We Just Copy? Cost-Sharing Arrangements and Characteristics of Health Care Systems," *Health Policy* 52.3 (2000): 11.
48. Ibid.
49. Jean-Pierre Poullier and Simone Sandier, "France," *Journal of Health Politics, Policy, and Law* 25.5 (2000): 899.
50. Ibid., 902.
51. Engelbert Theurl, "Some Aspects of the Reform of the Health Care Systems in Austria, Germany, and Switzerland," *Health Care Analysis* 7.4 (1999): 341.
52. Delnoij et al., "All Rights Reserved," 11.
53. Annette Tuffs, "Germany Expects More Hospital Privatization," *British Medical Journal* 320 (2000): 1030.
54. Delnoij et al., "All Rights Reserved," 11.
55. Miriam Wiley, "Ireland," *Journal of Health Politics, Policy, and Law* 25.5 (2000): 921.
56. Ibid.
57. Revital Gross, Bruse Rosen, and Arie Shirom, "Reforming the Israeli Health Care System: Findings of a 3-Year Evaluation," *Health Policy* 56.1 (2000): 11.
58. Ibid.
59. Delnoij et al., "All Rights Reserved," 12.
60. Peter Zweifel, "Switzerland," *Journal of Health Politics, Policy, and Law* 25.5 (2000): 939.
61. Delnoij et al., "All Rights Reserved," 12.
62. Betsy Powell, "'Passionate' Polly Leads Stars in Bid to Save Ontario's Medicare," *Toronto Star*, 23 May 01, A1.

MAKING HEALTH SPENDING WORK

Fred McMahon and Martin Zelder

"There is one certainty in this game: We're going to spend more money." So suggested a politician about the future of health care in a conversation. If recent history is any guide, this statement will prove accurate. Health spending is up dramatically, topping 22 percent in the last three years. Despite the recent and continuing surge in funding, waiting lists continue to grow. Why the disconnect? In this essay, economists Fred McMahon and Martin Zelder explain why greater funding does not result in higher quality.

"Consumers consume all the medical care they wish without regard for cost. Providers have incentives to boost their remuneration as much as possible without regard for either cost or quality of service." The two principle participants thus have little incentive to behave in the best interest of the system. "Only the bill paying bureaucracy has incentives to limit costs and create new efficiencies, but the distant bureaucracy can hardly match the inventiveness and on-the-spot knowledge of consumers and producers, who have no incentives to create new efficiencies and savings and who can often gain from waste and inefficiency."

These dynamics are a direct result of the command-and-control structure of medicare. They also have a detrimental impact on care: "This system lacks mechanisms to balance supply with demand. Queues and shortages become tools to control demand to fit the government-managed level of inadequate supply."

Moreover, economists McMahon and Zelder note the profound politicization of decision-making. Drawing on data from the 1990s, they note that the most effective health spending to reduce waiting lists is in the areas of pharmaceuticals and capital spending. And yet, "Only 1¢ of each new dollar entering the medicare system went to pharmaceuticals. Capital spending received only 2¢."

Instead of attempting to micromanage health care further, Martin and Zelder suggest an alternative: introducing market dynamics into the public system. In particular, they advocate medical savings accounts (MSAs). Under this proposal, the government would fund individuals, placing money into an account based on age, sex, and medical condition. People would then draw from these accounts to pay for basic medical services. Beyond a certain point, they would be covered by catastrophic insurance. In order to reward better spending, individuals would retain part of the balance at year's end.

MSAs would serve not simply as a demand management tool, though drawing from several studies, Martin and Zelder suggest this would be reason enough to support the idea; MSAs would go a step further, to liberate the supply side of the equation. By literally empowering people with health dollars, providers would compete and innovate to attract patients.

Introduction

The debate over Canadian health policy is curiously limited. Rather than applying the rich lessons derived from economic analysis,[1] most of those who debate health policy reform ignore market-based ideas, and instead focus almost exclusively on proposals that maintain the status quo, with only a few minor changes at the fringes of the system. In particular, the focus of debate is on supply, but through a command-and-control lens. Thus, debate centres on how to limit supply, or on the importance of devoting more tax dollars to increase supply, or on how to manage and administer better within the public system. What these narrow approaches share is an assumption that reform is best achieved through more extensive government control.

This essay contrasts the flaws and destructive incentives in medicare's current command-and-control structure with innovative ideas for the creation of a dramatically new and innovative system — a system with the potential to bring the benefits of market dynamics to the medical sector while maintaining the publicly funded nature of the system.

By ignoring market-based reforms and concentrating on centralized solutions, the present debate deprives Canadian citizens of the quality-of-life improvements they have realized in market-driven sectors — such as consumer goods, communications, entertainment, and so on — which dominate the rest of the economy. In those markets, the dynamic interaction of value-seeking consumers and competitive producers has led to huge gains for ordinary citizens. Hence, it is mind-boggling that we continue to view health policy reform in such a narrow and bureaucratic fashion.

This predisposition to seek governmental solutions to health policy problems was undoubtedly a by-product, originally, of Canadian compassion: low-income individuals should not be denied crucial medical care because of inability to pay. Unfortunately, this compassionate intent has not been well served by the institution of medicare. Preferential access to cardiovascular surgery on the basis of "nonclinical factors," such as personal prominence or political connections, is common.[2] As well, residents of suburban Toronto and Vancouver have longer waiting times than do their urban counterparts,[3] and residents of northern Ontario receive substantially lower travel reimbursement from the provincial government than do southern Ontarians when travelling for radiation treatment.[4] Finally, low-income Canadians are less likely to visit medical specialists,[5] including cardiac specialists, and have lower cardiac and cancer survival rates.[6]

The failure of this egalitarian dream is not medicare's only shortcoming. It is also, of course, grossly inefficient. This inefficiency is evidenced by prolonged and growing waiting times for care, discussed later in this essay. Moreover, the extent of the inefficiency is demonstrated by shocking new findings regarding the impact on health spending.

In this essay, we first examine the impact of medicare's current structure and the perverse incentives that arise from that structure. Then we explore a policy solution that creates market mechanisms even within a publicly funded system. We then turn to the impact of this policy solution on the health system's incentive structure and what this would mean for costs, productivity, allocative efficiency, demand patterns, and individual choice. We conclude with a brief discussion of some political considerations.

A House Divided

Medicare is a house divided against itself. Incentives facing the players in the system clash. Consumers consume all the medical care they wish without regard for cost. Providers have incentives to boost their remuneration as much as possible without regard for either cost or quality of service. Only the bill-paying bureaucracy has incentives to limit costs and create new efficiencies, but the distant bureaucracy can hardly match the inventiveness and on-the-spot knowledge of consumers and producers, who have no incentives to create new efficiencies and savings and who can often gain from waste and inefficiency.

Compare this scenario with a market system and how it aligns incentives. Consumers, because they are paying their own bills, have incentives to seek the most cost-efficient, quality services available. Providers' incentives are suddenly aligned with consumers' incentives. To gain customers, providers must compete to provide what consumers want: the most cost-efficient, high-quality services possible. The price signal moves resources to their most efficient allocation.

These dynamics create a stark contrast with medicare's command-and-control system. This system lacks mechanisms to balance supply with demand. Queues and shortages become tools to control demand to fit the government-managed level of inadequate supply. The system has no mechanisms to promote cost-efficient and high-quality services other than through bureaucratic fiat. Allocation is also determined by bureaucratic fiat, but without the information created by the price signal or with the knowledge of on-the-spot participants.

In a market, allocation of scarce resources is determined through the interaction of consumers and providers, which creates the price signal and a considerable amount of information. For instance, in a market-oriented system, a hospital would decide to buy an MRI machine based on whether usage justified the cost, rather than waiting for the decision of a health bureaucrat on allocation.

Let's consider in more depth the incentives facing consumers. While publicly insured medical services are, of course, not "free," but are financed by taxation, they are "free" in the important sense that they require no out-of-pocket payment by consumers at the time of use.[7] It is well known by economists everywhere that "free" services will be overused. Specifically, Newhouse and associates at the RAND think tank, in their pioneering and celebrated RAND Health Insurance Experiment, discovered that an insurance plan with modest out-of-pocket payments (compared with a plan with "free" care like Canada's) significantly reduced use of health care without impairing the health of participants, except for a small subgroup, poor participants with a serious medical condition like high blood pressure.[8] In other words, despite the paternalistic approach of Canada's medicare system, consumers are able to make their own choices. Only a small minority in special circumstances faces constraints that prevent this power to choose. Our proposal for a market-based medical system will have mechanisms to address this problem.

Now, contemplate the incentives for providers. They face prices for their publicly insured services that are centrally determined, via bargaining for doctors, nurses, and other health care workers. Because these prices are not the result of a market mechanism, it is unlikely that they correspond to the value to society of the underlying services. As a result, the level of services provided will not correspond to the level that society prefers. Additionally, hospitals are constrained by their government-determined budgets, mandates as to the numbers of treatments they can provide, and by their inability to receive financial rewards for serving consumers better.

Consequently, the outcome we observe in Canadian health care is one in which neither consumers nor providers are motivated to make desirable decisions. Consumers' lack of out-of-pocket responsibility leads them to demand some services with very low medical value. Doctors, nurses, and other health care professionals are not appropriately rewarded for what they do, and thus, justifiably, do not provide as many services as the public desires. Hospitals do not effectively compete because they are not rewarded for doing so. The taxpayers cover the costs of this misaligned system, relying on their agent — the government — to generate better results.

How well does the government do on our behalf? The traditional idealized view of the public-spirited bureaucrat has, in the last forty years, given way to a more realistic conception of government officials as self-interested creatures. As such, their decisions, like anybody else's, are aimed at achieving their own individual goals. But unlike Adam Smith's invisible hand, where the interaction of self-interested parties frequently leads to mutual benefit, the visible hand guiding government decision-makers often leads to an inefficient outcome. In such a state of affairs, the gains from reform exceed the costs, but reform still does not occur.

The reason that desirable reforms are not realized is because they are blocked by interest groups who can deliver a more appealing package of votes and financial support than the diffuse citizenry of taxpayers. For instance, public sector unions fight to maintain their virtual monopoly on staffing health facilities and the inflated wages that result from this monopoly situation. Their battle against privately managed clinics has nothing to do with promoting the health of Canadians and everything to do with politics and protecting union power. But surely superior health care should be the goal of medicare.

The inefficiency generated by political self-interest is manifested on a daily basis. Imagine that some set of hospital services could be best provided by private contractors, who use the government's fee schedule and bill the government so that service remains "free" to the consumer. This approach would make sense. Various forms of contracting out and privatization, usually introduced only after intense opposition from the bureaucracy, have brought great efficiencies to government.[9] Yet bureaucrats and politicians — along with public sector unions — have incentives to oppose private providers because private providers jeopardize their current arrangements and the privileges, power, and financial rewards associated with these arrangements. In short, the system creates incentives for small groups to frustrate attempts to improve the system for the benefit of average Canadians who need health care. Such conflicts are prevalent in matters small and large in the medicare system.

Of course, the incentive for self-interest runs through all human dealings. A for-profit hospital has every incentive to promote its services. But in a marketplace where choices are available, a hospital only attracts patients if it offers superior service or price, or both. However, in a public health care monopoly, consumers are left with no choice and must accept service where they can get it, regardless of quality.

Thus, consumer choices, distorted by medicare's insurance coverage and thwarted by a lack of serious options, combined with the decisions of self-interested politicians, lead to the systemic outcomes we observe. Crucial medical treatments are either denied consumers or — equally unfortunate — are not provided in a timely manner. Indeed, the most prominent evidence of the Canadian system's dysfunction is the prolonged and growing waiting time for treatment. Between 1993 and 1999, waiting time between a general practitioner's referral and treatment by a specialist rose from 9.3 to 14 weeks, a growth of 51 percent. Waiting times also rose dramatically for many critical types of care over this period, including medical oncology (114 percent), radiation oncology (65 percent), neurosurgery (43 percent), and orthopedic surgery (26 percent).[10]

Furthermore, Canada's record regarding waiting time is dismal when compared with other developed countries. In one study, Canadians waited longer than Americans for cranial MRI (5 months vs. 3 days), screening colonoscopy (4 weeks vs. 2 weeks), and total knee replacement (5.5 months vs. 3.5 weeks).[11] In another, Canadians waited longer than Germans and Americans respectively for cardiac catheterization (2.2 months vs. 1.7 months vs. 0 months), angioplasty (11 weeks vs. 7 weeks vs. 0 weeks), and bypass surgery (5.5 months vs. 4.4 months vs. 0 months).[12] A third study found that Canadians waited longer than Swedes and Americans for elective bypass surgery and urgent bypass surgery.[13]

The question then arises whether these waits are caused by flaws in the command-and-control system or by simple lack of resources. It is impossible to completely disentangle these two possibilities, but the evidence strongly points to the type of system flaws discussed in this essay. Public choice theory suggests that resources put into a public system will be disproportionately diverted to interest groups and administration.

Once again, consider incentives. Medical consumers are not allowed meaningful choices outside the government system. Thus, those working within the system — unlike those who work in a market-oriented sector — face no threat to their job or income if consumers are unsatisfied, since consumers can't take their business elsewhere. In fact, consumer dissatisfaction provides a rationale for demanding more money. Similarly, those working in the medicare system don't gain additional job security or pay raises if consumers are satisfied.

This means that those running the public health system have little incentive to actually improve services, but they do have immense incentives to build administrative structures and reward themselves as new resources enter the stream. The data is entirely consistent with this hypothesis. A comprehensive review of the relationship between spending and services discovered some startling relationships.[14]

Untargeted increases in health spending fail to reduce waiting times, except in Quebec. In fact, increases in spending are related to *increases* in waiting times for medical oncology, radiation oncology, and cardiovascular surgery. Additional spending also has no impact on the number of treatments offered by the medicare system. In a number of areas, higher spending is actually related to a *reduced* number of treatments. Such areas include total surgeries and radiology procedures.

These findings are consistent with public choice theory, which would predict that in a system like medicare, monies targeted to improve health care leak out to special interests. The theory would also predict that these special interests would devote much effort to capturing new monies, effort diverted from the actual provision of health care services. The system loses

twice, once through the capture of new income streams for special interests and again through the efforts expended to capture the income. Compare this system again with a market system where providers are penalized
when they divert resources to inefficient uses, as this action inhibits their
ability to meet demand from customers for cost-efficient, quality services.

The distribution of new dollars injected into the medicare system nicely
illustrates these points. Zelder found that expenditures on prescription
drugs reduced waiting times.[15] Capital spending also had positive benefits.
Zelder found it increased the number of procedures that health providers
are able to supply. Thus, in any rational system, one would expect new
spending to be heavily weighted to prescription drugs and capital spending. Public choice theory, however, would predict that little money would
go to drugs and capital spending since these expenditures go to outside
providers — pharmaceutical companies, pharmaceutical distributors and
retailers, building contractors, and equipment suppliers. Public choice
theory proves right: only 1¢ of each new dollar entering the medicare system
went to pharmaceuticals; capital spending received only 2¢.

Public choice theory would also predict that "insiders" would capture
most of the new money, even if that meant directing it to areas that provide little improvement in health care. This also proves to be correct. Out
of each dollar of new money, hospitals received 29¢, the catch-all category
"other" received 25¢, and "other institutions" received 23¢. This diversion of
resources almost certainly explains why increased spending is so ineffective
in improving medical services. Medicare promotes rent seeking that diverts
resources from medical care into the pockets of powerful special interest
groups, such as public sector unions.

Moreover, even administrators with the best of all intentions would face
an impossible task in running medicare. A distant bill-paying bureaucracy
simply does not have the tools or the information to control each medicare
transaction to promote efficiencies and savings. By contrast, in competitive market transactions, a party greatly interested in cost and quality —
the consumer — is present at every transaction. Providers compete to offer
the best service at the lowest cost.

Bureaucratic Responses

The bureaucratic response to medicare's problems is perverse. Rather than
opening up the system, empowering frontline providers, and expanding

choice, the bureaucracy has striven to tighten its control. Central bureaucracies decide which populations hospitals service, where hospitals are built, what treatments they provide and in what quantity, what equipment they buy, how much they can pay in salaries, what job descriptions are, and so on. As Canadian governments attempted to control the growth of medical care costs, they typically put a centralized bureaucracy or special planning commission in charge of making the difficult decisions about retrenchment.

For example, the Ontario Health Care Restructuring Commission, in its report on hospitals, made recommendations from the large-scale (which hospitals would be closed and which left open) to the small-scale (which wards in individual hospitals would be shut down, how many beds would be closed, and which services individual hospitals would no longer provide). The government of Ontario then acted on the bulk of the recommendations.

Government is now laying siege to the remaining outposts of independence: federal Health Minister Allan Rock has declared he likes the proposal from Ontario's Restructuring Commission to force all family physicians into group practices, where the bureaucracy would have the power to micromanage down to the last receptionist's salary. Fierce opposition from doctors forced the Ontario government to back away from the most coercive measures recommended by the commission, but governments across Canada — including the federal government — continue to discuss ways to increase government control over doctors' practices and the provision of medical services.

Similar perversities are found on the demand side. Demand is matched to supply not by the price signal — the most efficient system of allocation and production in human history — but rather through queues, rules, and rationing. Each can produce absurd, and sometimes tragic, results.

Internal Dysfunction

A particularly severe area of dysfunction in the system is the human resource sector. While markets match staffing demands with labour supply through the price signal — whether at the level of vice-president or janitor — in the medicare system, pay structures are determined by centralized processes, which are sensitive to politics and the power of various groups. With rare exceptions, individuals are not permitted to form contracts at mutually agreed upon prices, so groups must bargain collectively, which inevitably serves Canada's unions.

278 • BETTER MEDICINE

The health care bureaucracies have been careful to protect their monopoly employment power within each province by, among other things, effectively limiting consumer choices in the provision of medical services to providers within the medicare system. This protection has been accomplished by laws that place restrictive conditions on physicians wishing to opt out of the public system, and require provincial licensing of private hospitals. Of course, the expanded choice provided by opted-out doctors and private hospitals would undermine the system's monopoly if consumers decided the private providers offered better services. Hence, political pressure by interest groups (e.g., public sector unions) has discouraged such private sector developments.

Moreover, political competition among provincial medical associations, nurses' unions, and other health sector unions has created a system in which pay is not clearly linked to social value. This politicized, government-bargained process leads to perverse salary decisions within the system. Power, and more importantly, the willingness to use it, drives remuneration levels. All of this adds up to a bizarre health care system in which medical workers are underpaid and nonmedical staff is overpaid. One indication of this imbalance is the relative compensation of physicians, nurses, and other medical workers. Although a direct determination of occupational value is difficult, one can gain a sense of the appropriateness of compensation by comparing data from the Organisation for Economic Co-Operation and Development (OECD) on Canadian and U.S. incomes. This comparison reveals that while Canadian physicians earn only 50 percent of what U.S. physicians do, Canadian nurses earn 85 percent of their American counterparts' average, and "all medical workers" on average earn 93 percent, in Canada, of the U.S. average.[16] Because doctors and nurses are included in the "medical workers" calculation, this means that those medical workers who are neither doctors nor nurses (i.e., technicians, plus those in nonmedical jobs such as hospital janitors) earn more than 93 percent of their U.S. counterparts, perhaps 100 percent, perhaps more!

Political power is a likely explanation of this perverse salary structure. Doctors may be reluctant to strike. Many entered the health care profession because of a strong commitment to caring and medicine. Thus, doctors may hesitate to withhold services. In a publicly administered compensation system, where power largely determines pay levels, government can play hardball with doctors because their resolve to strike is weak. This tendency is reflected in a comment by New Brunswick Premier Bernard Lord during the New Brunswick doctors' strike in early 2001: "Do they want to take the patients of New Brunswick hostage? Is that their objective?" Because of such rhetoric, and because of the weakness of physicians' bargaining tactics, their strikes are often short-lived. In their recent dispute, New Brunswick doctors gave up their strike after three days, without any settlement or even much movement on the government's side, despite the fact that their fees are 30 percent less, on average, than those of doctors in neighbouring Nova Scotia.[17]

This kind of situation has enabled government's health care bureaucracy to shift much of the burden of the financial squeeze medicare has suffered in recent years onto the backs of doctors and nurses. That both professions are being underpaid is evident in the shortages of doctors and nurses that have developed from coast to coast. It is also evident in the permanent immigration flows between Canada and the U.S. Over the 1980–97 period, about fifteen nurses left Canada for the U.S. for every one who entered. Over the same period, about nineteen doctors left Canada for the U.S. for every one who entered.[18] However, Canada suffers no shortage of well-paid, unionized nonmedical workers in the medical system. Demonstrating the perversity of the current system, medicare promotes underpay for and shortages of health workers in the health system, while at the same time promoting overpay for nonmedical workers.

The press loves to trumpet the stories about doctors who earn an obscene amount of money, and some do abuse the system. As of 1995, the average GP (general practitioner), after the considerable expenses of running an office, earns just under $100,000 in annual income.[19] But Statistics Canada reports that doctors, on average, work 40 percent more hours than a typical Canadian. So if a doctor worked an average number of hours, that pay packet is reduced to just over $70,000 a year.

Moreover, family doctors in private practice do not receive fringe benefits. They fund their own pensions, provide their own disability insurance, insure their spouses and children, etc. The cost of benefit packages varies considerably, but a conservative estimate is that they are worth about 20 percent of the base salary. This means that a doctor who worked about as many hours as the average Canadian would pull in a pay rate equivalent of about $56,000 a year. That's less than an experienced teacher or autoworker earns. It is far less than the earnings of many people who hold skilled or semiskilled jobs, which don't require a university education and years of lost earning power.

However, nonmedical workers in the health care system receive a golden harvest. For example, while New Brunswick doctors returned to work without a settlement, the government of New Brunswick broke its own wage guidelines in its offer to hospital workers, represented by the Canadian Union of Public Employees (CUPE). Even so, the government had to threaten to legislate CUPE back to work. That action outraged militant unionists, who had been prepared to use their strike power regardless of the health care consequences. CUPE gave in to the legislative threat, but not without warnings of revenge from CUPE president Judy Darcy. The government, she said, would be "confronted by the full force of the labour movement." [20]

This kind of threat gets the attention of politicians and bureaucrats. One study of hospital pay levels in British Columbia found that unionized nonmedical hospital workers (e.g., janitors), depending on their job type, receive 25 to 63 percent more in pay than those doing the same job in the private sector.[21] It is not surprising, then, that CUPE has funded and organized the fight against allowing private providers in the public system.

Yet in Canada's often bizarre medicare debate, even supposedly expert commentators frequently mangle reality. For example, *Financial Post* columnist Linda McQuaig writes that "doctors enjoy enormous political clout. Politicians who seem to welcome a good fight with public sector janitors and clerical staff tend to shy away from getting into fights with people they're likely to run into later at the golf club."[22] But why would Canada be suffering shortages of doctors if governments so quickly caved in to their demands? Why would CUPE be able to fight so successfully against any reform to allow private providers if government was so willing to beat up on "janitors and clerical staff," as McQuaig has it? Surely, these workers would be the first to demand a liberalization of the medicare system if their government pay was suffering in comparison with pay in the private sector.

By contrast, in early 2001, when Alberta gave its doctors a significant fee increase, health officials across Canada reacted with public condemnation.[23] There should be no competition for doctors, the officials appeared to be saying. Of course, without effective competition to pay doctors what they are worth in Canada, capable doctors will increasingly migrate to the United States, and other qualified young people will pass on the prospect of medical school. At this rate, hospitals may soon be full of well-paid janitors and cooks, but devoid of doctors and nurses.

Introducing Market Dynamics to Publicly Funded Health Care

Markets eliminate the twisted incentives of a bureaucratic system. The consumer becomes the bill payer, pursuing the very simple objective of getting the best possible result at the least possible cost. To succeed, providers must meet the consumer demand for cost-efficient service. The incentives of all the players in the system now lead to the same goal: improved efficiencies and reduced costs. The price signal balances supply with demand.

Yet in Canada's current medicare debate, it's usually assumed that market dynamics cannot be grafted onto publicly funded medicare, even though policy innovations have successfully used market mechanisms to achieve public ends in other areas — charter schools and school vouchers, tradable pollution rights, and property rights to promote conservation in the fishery, for example.

Medical savings accounts (MSAs) have the potential to bring market dynamics to a publicly funded medicare system. Under an MSA scheme, the government funds an MSA for each family or individual. The family or individual then draws on the MSA to pay for medical services. This empowers the consumer by providing choice.[24] MSAs can be structured in a number of different ways. Consider one possible scheme: Each year the government funds a personalized MSA for every Canadian. Projected medical expenses, based on factors such as age, sex, and medical condition, determine the amount paid into the MSA. The MSA can only be spent on a designated list of health services, which could include not only currently insured services, but items not currently insured, such as dental care, vision care, and alternative medicine. Those who spend less than their allotted amount during the year may retain some or all of the balance.

Those who exceed their allowance would be covered by an "overcharge" fund, roughly equivalent to catastrophic health insurance, but designed to cover medical expenses which, for whatever reason, exceed the individual's MSA. Affluent Canadians could be made responsible for paying some costs on their own before accessing the fund. The fund would kick in immediately for poorer Canadians, so they would never be charged for medical services. This would remedy the problem the RAND study, discussed earlier, found for some groups of poor patients.

MSAs are usually thought of as a demand management tool. MSAs give consumers a strong financial incentive to economize on their medicare consumption, a much better outcome than bureaucratically imposed

282 * BETTER MEDICINE

queues, rules, and rationing, which cannot account for differing situations or preferences. A great deal of evidence has recently been accumulated regarding the desirable effects of MSAs. A 1996 RAND study found that if all insured nonelderly Americans switched to MSAs, their health spending would decline by at least 6 and as much as 13 percent.[25] But although MSAs are not widespread in the U.S., due to severe regulatory restrictions on their structure,[26] they are the type of insurance held by 50 percent of South Africans.[27] In that setting, they have dramatically reduced health spending, including a reduction in outpatient spending by approximately 50 percent, as well as a reduction in inpatient spending.[28] Besides these cost savings, MSAs would individually benefit a substantial majority of the population, including those most prone to illness, according to a recent study from the Urban Institute.[29] The application of MSAs in the Canadian context has been described in Ramsay, Litow and Muller, and Gratzer.[30]

MSAs could also liberate the supply side of the medicare system. For example, centralized fee schedules bargained by governments should be abolished; as well, the provision of hospital services should be opened to all qualified providers, whether for-profit, not-for-profit, or public sector. Consumers should be able to choose among them based on normal consumer preferences such as cost, quality, and convenience.

With consumers paying their own health bills though their MSAs, along with these other supply-side reforms, health providers' incomes would be determined by revenue from MSAs rather than by bureaucratic fiat. This would allow the price signal to emerge and carry information through the system. Consumers would have an incentive to seek the most cost-effective care possible. Providers would be unleashed from bureaucratic control to meet this demand, and incentives would consequently be realigned to boost productivity and effective allocation of resources.

For example, central planning authorities previously have proved unable to provide enough MRI machines to the right hospitals, as is evidenced by long waits for MRIs in much of Canada. However, if a hospital were autonomous and able to buy its own MRI machines based on usage and a market-based fee schedule, it would be rewarded for providing the level of service demanded. In other words, each institute would have the incentive and the ability to provide the services needed in its community. A number of private clinics are now trying to meet the demand for MRIs that central planning has failed to fulfill, but the federal government says even this incentive violates the "spirit" of medicare.

Under the MSA system, efficiency occurs naturally, as part of the system dynamics. For instance, the Ontario Health Care Restructuring Commission's proposal to force all family doctors into group practices open twenty-four hours a day, seven days a week, was largely designed to reduce the use of emergency wards in off hours. But if consumers had been given an MSA-style incentive to minimize their health bill, and providers were able to receive rewards for providing demanded services, off-hour alternatives to emergency visits would undoubtedly now be commonplace.

The MSA concept is flexible and could fit into any number of structures. For instance, an MSA system could maintain a "one-tiered" health care system. Except for the buffer area between MSA coverage and "overcharge" coverage, which could be implemented for higher-income Canadians, health care providers could be prohibited from accepting private, non-MSA payment for health services, except for providers who opt out of the public system altogether and thus may not receive MSA payments. This scenario would be similar to the current system under which, for example, doctors may only bill the government for approved services.[31]

Political Dynamics

Public sector unions and the most dogmatic elements of Canada's left wing will oppose MSAs, as will those who believe individuals are not capable of making their own choices. Nonetheless, MSAs could have surprising political appeal for much of the Canadian political spectrum, in part because the Canadian public has been quicker than Canadian politicians to realize that the system needs reform. It is also in part because MSAs can be viewed favourably from both left-wing and right-wing positions.

Although many in the Canadian left, who remain attached to the idea of government management, will attack any reform, MSAs are in fact both a health policy and an income redistribution policy, something that should appeal to left-wing thinkers. General revenues will support MSAs, while an individual's MSA will be based on medical need, regardless of income. In fact, the idea behind MSAs might well be described as, "From each according to ability, to each according to need." According to surveys, it is low-income people who are most attracted by MSAs.[32]

As for the right, MSAs can be presented as similar to tax breaks, in that each individual receives an allowance he or she controls, although an MSA must be spent on health care and contains a redistributive aspect. Nonetheless, this situation is different from government absorbing the money, or spending it for you. It should also appeal because it employs market mechanisms.

Finally, MSAs are politically self-equilibrating. Individuals will directly know, from their MSA balances, when the system is being underfunded, creating pressure for governments to provide appropriate funding while generating support for such funding, particularly since people will see the funds flowing directly into their personal MSAs.

Conclusion

No Canadian should be deprived of standard medical care because of inability to pay. But Canada's health care sector need not remain a command-economy experiment. No civilized society should (or would) allow someone to die of an easily treatable medical condition because that person lacks the money to pay for care. Yet Canadians now die because they lack a properly structured health care system.

The answer is not more bureaucratic control. The answer is grafting the efficiency and dynamism of market economies onto our publicly funded system. An MSA system creates dynamics for gains in productivity, improved resource allocation, and sensible demand patterns. Even more importantly, it allows individuals to regain control of their own medical decisions and provides the choices needed for such control to become a reality.

NOTES

1. For more on health care and economics, see the essay by William Watson in this volume.
2. David A. Alter, Antoni S.H. Basinski, and C. David Naylor, "A Survey of Provider Experiences and Perceptions of Preferential Access to Cardiovascular Care in Ontario, Canada," *Annals of Internal Medicine* 129 (1998): 567–72.
3. Cynthia Ramsay, "Outside the City Walls: Not So Equal Access to Health Care in Canada," *Fraser Forum*, Jan. 1997, 19–23.
4. Lisa Priest, "Northern Ontario Cancer Patients Face 'Discrimination': Many complain that they must pay hotel, gas and other expenses that are covered for patients from southern Ontario who travel for treatment," *Globe and Mail*, 17 June 2000, A3.
5. Sheryl Dunlop, Peter C. Coyte, and Warren McIsaac, "Socio-Economic Status and the Utilisation of Physicians' Services: Results from the Canadian National Population Health Survey," *Social Science and Medicine*, 2000, 1–11.
6. David A. Alter, C. David Naylor, Peter Austin, and Jack V. Tu, "Effects of Socioeconomic Status on Access to Invasive Cardiac Procedures and on Mortality after Acute

Myocardial Infarction," *New England Journal of Medicine* 341 (1999): 1359–67 and W.J. Mackillop, J. Zhang-Salomons, P.A. Groome, L. Paszat, and E. Holowaty. "Socioeconomic Status and Cancer Survival in Ontario," *Journal of Clinical Oncology* 15 (1997): 1680–89.

7. Premiums are collected as well in British Columbia and Alberta.

8. Joseph P. Newhouse and the Insurance Experiment Group, *Free for All? Lessons from the RAND Health Insurance Experiment* (Cambridge: Harvard University Press, 1993).

9. The evidence for this efficiency in the hospital business is described in Martin Zelder, *How Private Hospital Competition Can Improve Canadian Health Care* (Vancouver: The Fraser Institute, 2000).

10. Martin Zelder, *Waiting Your Turn: Hospital Waiting Lists in Canada*, 10th ed. (Vancouver: The Fraser Institute, 2000) and Cynthia Ramsay and Michael Walker, *Waiting Your Turn: Hospital Waiting Lists in Canada*, 4th ed. (Vancouver: The Fraser Institute, 1994).

11. Chaim M. Bell, Matthew Crystal, Allan S. Detsky, and Donald A. Redelmeier, "Shopping Around for Hospital Services," *Journal of the American Medical Association* 279 (1998): 1015–17.

12. R.L. Collins-Nakai, H.A. Huysmans, and H.E. Scully, "Task Force 5: Access to Cardiovascular Care: An International Comparison," *Journal of the American College of Cardiology* 19 (1992): 1477–85.

13. R.J. Carroll, S.D. Horn, B. Soderfeldt, B.C. James, and L. Malmberg, "International Comparison of Waiting Times for Selected Cardiovascular Procedures," *Journal of the American College of Cardiology* 25 (1995): 557–63.

14. Martin Zelder, "The Myth of Underfunded Medicare in Canada," *Fraser Forum*, Aug. 2000, 1–48.

15. Martin Zelder, *How Private Hospital Competition Can Improve Canadian Health Care*.

16. The incomes compared are adjusted for differences in purchasing power, and are from the most recent year in which both Canadian and American figures are available: 1992 for MDs, 1986 for nurses, and 1995 for "all medical workers." See Organisation for Economic Co-Operation and Development (OECD), *Health Data*, electronic version, 2000.

17. "N.B. Doctors Going on Strike Next Week: Looking for 30 Percent Raise over Three Years," *Globe and Mail* Web site, 4 Jan. 2001.

18. Drew Murray and J. Zhao, "Brain Drain and Gain: Part I, The Emigration of Knowledge Workers from Canada," *Canadian Economic Observer* (Ottawa: Statistics Canada, 2000).

19. All of the data in this discussion of GP earnings are from Abdul Rashid, "Earnings of Physicians," *Perspectives on Labour and Income* 11 (1999): 27–38.

20. CUPE Web site, www.cupe.ca.

21. Cynthia Ramsay, "Labour Costs in the Hospital Sector," *Fraser Forum*, Nov. 1995, 16–18.

22. Linda McQuaig, "Let's Disempower Doctors," *National Post* Web site, 15 Jan. 2001.

23. Larry Johnsrude, "Provinces Fear New Battle for MDs After Alberta Deal," *National Post* Web site, 30 Jan. 2001.

24. Lawrence Solomon, "Patients, Heal Thyselves!" *Nextcity*, Fall 1996.

25. Emmet B. Keeler, J. D. Malkin, D. P. Goldman, and J. L. Buchanan, "Can Medical Savings Accounts for the Nonelderly Reduce Health Care Costs?" *Journal of the American Medical Association* 275 (1996): 1666–71.

26. Greg Scandlen, "Four Years of MSAs: The Lessons So Far." *Brief Analysis No. 327* (Dallas: National Center for Policy Analysis, 2000).

27. Shaun Matisonn, "Medical Savings Accounts in South Africa," *Policy Report No. 234* (Dallas: National Center for Policy Analysis, 2000).

28. Ibid.

29. Len M. Nichols, Marilyn Moon, and Susan Wall, "Tax-Preferred Medical Savings Accounts and Catastrophic Health Insurance Plans: A Numerical Analysis of Winners and Losers," manuscript, The Urban Institute, 1996.

30. See Cynthia Ramsay, *Medical Savings Accounts: Universal, Accessible, Portable, Comprehensive Health Care for Canadians* (Vancouver: The Fraser Institute, 1998), Mark Litow and Stacy Muller, *Feasibility of Health Care Allowances in Canada*, prepared by Milliman & Robertson (Toronto: The Consumer Policy Institute, 1998), and David Gratzer, *Code Blue: Reviving Canada's Health Care System* (Toronto: ECW Press, 1999).

31. Whether it would be wise to create such restrictions is another question. The point here is simply that the MSA concept has adequate flexibility to meet such concerns.

32. Angus Reid Group, *Canadians' Perceptions of the Health Allowance System* (Toronto: The Consumer Policy Institute, 1997).

THE ABCs OF MSAs

David Gratzer

As frustration mounts with both the quality and timeliness of health care in Canada, a hunger for new ways of thinking has developed. Canadians, for the most part, are stuck listening to ideas of the spendthrifts ("Spend more money!") and the magicians ("Manage the system better with primary care reform and more home care!"). Both groups propose government solutions to the problem, leading to greater bureaucratic control over health delivery. In this essay, I propose the road not taken: a system built on individual choice and competition, through medical savings accounts (MSAs).

MSAs are based on three very simple principles. First, minor health expenses (what economists term "discretionary spending") are treated differently from major expenses (termed "catastrophic expenses"). Second, financial incentives exist to encourage people's frugality with minor expenses. And finally, insurance protects people against major expenses.

This essay looks at several experiments with the MSA concept. It begins by reviewing Singapore's health care system. Since 1984, Singapore has required citizens to save part of their income in a Medisave account, which is used for hospital care. Singapore public hospitals compete for patient funding with private institutions, resulting in what one health expert terms, "a very, very efficient system." Singapore boasts universal coverage, many more MRIs per capita than Canada, and a longer life expectancy while spending just a fraction of the GDP on health care.

While our health care system differs dramatically from U.S. medicine, in both countries, people don't pay directly for their health care. The result south of the border has been a proliferation of managed care plans. While Singapore's experiment is hospital-based, MSAs have also been used in the United States for all medical delivery, and are gaining popularity as an alternative to managed care. For employees of companies like Golden Rule, Quaker Oats, and Jersey City, MSAs have meant greater control over their health care; for the employers, there is also the bonus of cost savings.

In South Africa, MSAs have grown to become the most popular form of private insurance, covering some 4.6 million people. The experiment originated in the Mandela government's decision to deregulate the health insurance market, in part to reduce the load on the public system. Insurers have noted that MSAs cut noncatastrophic expenses by roughly 50 percent. In China, an MSA-based concept was introduced to cover people in different urban centres in an attempt to achieve cost control. It did — health costs have fallen.

These experiments differ greatly among jurisdictions, from the insurance policies purchased by American firms for their employees to Chinese government-financed plans for their citizens. Regardless of the nature of the experimentation, the basic result is similar: patient empowerment and cost savings. As the troubles with our system grow it's worth considering MSAs, which could well provide universal health care without our present malaise.

Walking into the corporate headquarters of Destiny Health, it's difficult not to feel that the office is very American. To be sure, the small insurance company doesn't boast a lavish or particularly well-decorated headquarters. There are no Americana paintings on the wall or flags in the corners. And the receptionist doesn't once make reference to the Founding Fathers when she offers me coffee.

Maybe it's the location. Destiny Health's office is a twenty-minute drive from the White House, just over the Maryland border. The drive itself is largely on big American interstate highways with their cryptic numberings.

Whatever the reason, I feel the American environment as I wait. Finally, CEO Ken Linde greets me. After a quick handshake, he escorts me into his office. We sit and chat about health care. Or, more correctly, he talks.

Linde describes his company and its product in an all-encompassing monologue. He touches on the evolution of the health insurance industry in the United States, the implications of aging demographics on American medicine, and the federal surplus. And he goes on; he critiques car insurance, describes his wife's retirement benefit package, details his daughter's job. The flow breaks once when he pops out of his chair to grab a company pamphlet. The monologue is exhaustive and exhausting. It is, effectively, a sales pitch.

The terminology itself is unfamiliar to a Canadian: patients are "customers," health coverage is an "insurance." Even Linde's basic approach to health care is so very different from what we're accustomed to in Canada. There is no talk about quality care, home care, or any of the other topics that dominate our discussions. Instead, Linde talks about his company's "package" and business opportunities leading to expansion.

It is all very American: sitting in an American office, listening to an American CEO outline his company's most American of activities, receiving the glib American sales pitch. The irony, of course, is that while Linde is American, his company is not. Destiny Health is a subsidiary of Discovery Health of South Africa. Indeed, the product Linde sells as the next step in the evolution of the U.S. health market is, he confesses, a "retinkered" version of the policy sold by his parent company an ocean away. That policy, a type of medical savings account (MSA), is the number one–selling private health insurance in South Africa.

Much of our health care debate in Canada is internally focused. When we do discuss alternatives to the present structure of medicare, the conversation shifts south. As noted in David Henderson's essay in this volume, many of our perceptions of the American system are incorrect. But a bigger mistake that Canadians make is assuming that the choice for reform is between an inefficient but universal system, and an efficient but nonuniversal one.

MSAs offer a method of preserving the universality of the present health care system with improved efficiency, patient-focus, and quality. This essay describes MSA experiments in several countries, beginning with Singapore. Along the way, I will discuss the problem with medicare's current structure and suggest possible models for Canadian MSAs. Finally, I will answer some basic questions about the MSA concept.

1. Singapore

Since the concept of medical savings accounts originated in this city-state, Singapore is a good place to start our discussion. Of course, it may seem like an odd choice: Singapore boasts a population smaller than Toronto's; it is nestled on a land mass that could comfortably fit onto Prince Edward Island. But in the unusual freedom-based concept of MSAs, the ultracontrol Singapore government may have found an effective way of delivering universal health care.

For the most part, descriptions of other health care systems tend to be reduced to numbers: infant mortality rates, physicians per capita, etc. Of course, those statistics are important, but understanding the Singapore system requires more than an overview of numbers. Singapore offers a health care system that seems very familiar in some respects and yet surprisingly alien. Singapore has a universal health care system featuring modern hospitals, state-of-the-art equipment, and well-trained physicians. Singapore has a health care system entirely built on individual choice, emphasizing competition and cost sharing.

Let's, then, consider a clinical scenario.

On a trip to Singapore, you feel pain in your abdomen. Initially, you shrug it off — it's probably just an upset stomach, you reason. But after a few days, as the pain grows stronger, you decide it's time to see a doctor. Indeed, you can barely stand up. This is an emergency, and so you head to an emergency room.

In Canada, there wouldn't be much in the way of making a decision: you'd head for a public hospital, of course. But in Singapore, you must choose, not simply among the institutions, but among the *types* of institutions. Unlike Canada, Singapore has no laws or regulations banning private hospitals. In fact, the government likes the presence of nonpublic hospitals because they increase the efficiency of all hospitals. You can thus head to Singapore General (government-owned) or Gleneagles (private) or a score of other choices, all of which are of assured quality since all hospitals conform to basic standards and physicians often hold cross-appointments.

As you approach Singapore General, you notice a sign for valet parking. In Singapore, patients pay for part of their care out of a Medisave account (more on this to follow). As a result, patients are *customers*. In most of Canada, hospital funding is divorced from patient load and satisfaction. In other words, patients are *users* of the health care system.

The difference is obvious. Singapore hospitals work hard at patient satisfaction: emergency rooms post waiting times (and keep them minimal), hospitals are clean and the food is edible, most facilities offer valet parking. Feedback is important: patient surveys literally litter the waiting rooms.

Of course, as you enter into Accident and Emergency (A&E), valet parking isn't the biggest issue on your mind. Holding your aching tummy, you immediately approach the triage desk. As you walk through the waiting area, you may feel you're in a Canadian hospital: you find people hurrying around, you hear the rattle of printers, and you observe people talking. About forty patients sit in the waiting area. A posted sign suggests that your waiting time will be an hour.

That's a bit unusual for Singapore. Most ERs see patients quickly. After all, a dissatisfied patient is unlikely to return. In fact, many hospitals brag that patients are seen, as a rule, within fifteen minutes (compare that with the long waits Canadians face).[1]

Given the gravity of the situation, you are quickly triaged and prioritized. Soon, you are lying on a bed waiting for the physician, who arrives carrying your chart and proceeds with a history and physical. Because any number of problems can cause abdominal pain, some blood tests are ordered and you are sent for an X-ray. When these tests prove inconclusive, it's suggested you undergo a CT scan.

CT scans are hard to get in Canada. Even in emergency situations (including strokes and head trauma) the wait can be hours in an ER, even if the facility has a scanner. But in Singapore, there is plenty of diagnostic machinery. In fact, there are many more CT scanners and MRIs per capita than in Canada. Even getting an outpatient test is fast — patients typically wait a day or two for an MRI scan. By contrast, a study found that Canadians wait on average 150 days for an MRI.

In less than an hour, you are wheeled down for the picture. After the test, the physician comes back and shares some diagnostic possibilities. It's not entirely clear, but it seems that you may have an inflammatory bowel disease, perhaps Chron's. You need more tests (including a scope) and a trial of steroids. Given all this, the doctor feels that an admission is called for.

In Canada, getting a bed in a hospital is no easy matter. Patients often wait hours, sometimes days. Fortunately for you, there will be no lengthy wait in Singapore. You'll be moved up to a ward — as soon as you choose one. Hospitals offer different types of wards, ranging from crowded to luxurious.

Remember, for Singapore citizens, the hospital fee comes out of a Medisave account. At the General, a bed on a Class C ward is under $100 a day. You would need to share the room with many others in this Victorian-style ward. Up on the more exclusive Class A ward, where rooms have but one bed, the cost is a stiffer $823 a day. For those who want something in between, there is Class B1 (three to four beds), B2+ (five beds), and B2 (six to ten beds). The physicians are the same on all the wards. The difference in price, then, is due to cost and government subsidies. Those less able to pay are subsidized more, but stay in less posh accommodations.

And so begins your Singapore hospital stay.

What is a Medisave account? How does Singapore achieve universal care with choice? Is this really relevant to Canada? To answer these questions, let's consider the history of Singapore's health care system.

The bold health care experiment began, in fact, with pensions. Eager to encourage savings, the colonial government developed a state pension plan in 1955 not unlike the Canada Pension Plan: with contributions from both workers and employers, people could save for their retirement and draw from the plan starting at age fifty-five. The original contribution was set at 5 percent of income, matched by employers.[2]

Soon after independence, the savings account idea — known as the Central Provident Fund — was revisited. Workers simply couldn't save enough with the arrangement. The plan, in other words, was elegant and simple, but inadequate.

The Singapore government soon required greater savings. To capitalize on compound interest so workers could enhance their retirement nest egg, the government also allowed limited investment in stocks and bonds. Over the years, the Central Provident Fund's role has been expanded to cover disability insurance, home downpayments, mortgage repayments, and college tuition. Workers, thus, had a super-RRSP.

And so Singapore developed its welfare state programs without a big, expensive government. As with so many other facets of life in Singapore, a Western observer will find much about bureaucracy that is familiar and yet much that isn't. The role the government has taken — involving itself in issues such as housing and retirement — is similar to the government's role in countries like Britain and Canada. The approach of using mandatory retirement savings — instead of large, bureaucratic, tax-financed programs — is unique, however. Home ownership soared (and is, per capita, the highest in the world) even though there has been a limited subsidization in public housing; retirement monies accrued without a state-run pension plan; and college became accessible despite modest loan programs.

Singapore's compulsory savings resulted in huge capital resources for a relatively small country, helping pay for its infrastructure and its explosive growth. When granted independence in 1965, no one assumed this former colonial trading post would survive; today, the country boasts the fourth largest economy in the world.

Of course, medical insurance was missing from any government experimentation. As the "high-tech, high-expense" medical revolution reshaped health care, the Singapore government looked abroad for answers.

What they saw was more welfare statism. In Britain, the Labour government moved to cover all citizens in the late 1940s. Impressed with the British National Health Service (NHS), every Canadian province had joined a national plan by the early 1970s. Singapore, however, resisted the trend. Within the government, various ideas were debated. Many were impressed by the approach of countries like Britain and Canada. Others, however, were more restrained and eventually won out, implementing a distinctly Singaporean solution to the health care issue.[3] In 1984, Singapore's government expanded the system of mandatory savings to cover health care. Now, each worker is required to put a certain percentage of his or her income in a tax-free account, known as a Medisave account.

The account's monies are meant to cover hospital expenses, not outpatient treatment. Thus, a trip to the family doctor with a sprained ankle is not a Medisave expense. (Most outpatient services are either partially subsidized and offered in government clinics or are privately financed.) A hospital stay, be it one day or three months, is a Medisave expense.

There are many problems with the Singapore system. A government that feels its role includes banning spitting in public has no hesitation engaging in a bit of health care social engineering. Feminists beware: medical school admission policies discriminate against women with the justification that men — free from child rearing — work longer hours.

But it's difficult not to admire some aspects of the system.[4] Singapore boasts more diagnostic machinery than Canada. Physician compensation is better in the city-state relative to average wages, while length-of-hospital-stays stats are comparable. Infant mortality is lower in Singapore. Life expectancy is modestly longer than here. Emergency room overcrowding is rare. Waiting lists for surgeries are minimal.

Tricia Edmonds from Vancouver isn't an expert on health care. She doesn't quote statistics or discuss economic principles. She offers instead a simple comparison, based on her own experience as a patient. In 1996, she delivered a baby in Singapore after a difficult pregnancy. She has also given birth in Canada. "If I ran into problems, I'd rather be in a Singapore hospital," she states bluntly. "The care was excellent."[5]

Earlier in this volume, health economist Cynthia Ramsay describes the findings of her major international health system comparison. Singapore tops the United States and Britain — and Canada. That's not bad considering that health spending in Singapore is under 4 percent of GDP; in Canada, we spend between 9 and 10 percent.

Why does Singapore do so well? "The whole idea of personal responsibility for health care is important," notes Ramsay. "People also have more choice — they can go to a private hospital or a public hospital, they choose among different wards. In other words, they shop around. Online, Singapore citizens have access to information on waiting times and quality. Citizens have to be educated — and they are."[6]

There are other points to critique, but to do so may not be fair. Singapore doesn't claim to have a perfect health care system. But the Singapore approach is very unusual in that it values individual choice and competition.

This fact may not seem particularly significant except that it flies in the face of our entire approach. In Canada, heath care is effectively a government monopoly. And, as with all monopolies, the result is a costly system with little concern for patient convenience or satisfaction. Singapore also has universal health care, but patients partly fund the system with their Medisave accounts. Accountability, streamlined administration, and timely care are the result.

Dr. Thomas Massaro is a pediatrician with Virginia State Hospital. He is also an expert on health administration, having published numerous papers on the subject. On Singapore health care, Dr. Massaro says simply, "It's a very, very efficient system."[7]

No wonder, then, that countries as a diverse as the United States and China have found something of value in the Singapore experience.

2. What Happened to Medicare?

Before discussing other MSA experiments around the world, let's pause and ask the relevant question: What happened to Canada's health care system?

This volume, particularly Part 1, documents many of the problems with which Canadians are well familiar: declining standards in care, signalled by the long waiting times for practically any diagnostic test or treatment; overcrowding in the ERs; scraping by with limited equipment. This dire situation has developed despite increases in spending and aggressive administrative reforms.

But why is medicare in decline? The answer stems from its structure. Medicare, after all, is supposed to be insurance. But if that was the goal, we overreached — medicare covers people in *every* situation.

Nobel laureate Milton Friedman summarizes the distortion of insurance:

We generally rely on insurance to protect us against events that are highly unlikely to occur but involve large losses if they do occur — major catastrophes, not minor regularly recurring expenses. We insure our houses against loss from fire, not against the cost of having to cut the lawn. We insure our cars against liability to others or major damage, not against having to pay for gasoline. Yet in medicine, it has become common to rely on insurance to pay for regular medical examinations and often for prescriptions.[8]

The distortion of health insurance has cost implications. Consider, to continue Friedman's example, if car insurance did cover gas. How much would you drive? Or what if your home insurance covered more than just fire and acts of God — house painting, window washing, recarpeting, wallpapering, and cleaning? Wouldn't you be tempted to paint the den a different colour every year?

And, indeed, by distorting the concept of health insurance, medicare changed the way people use health services and the way these services are provided. Simply put, medicare has corrupted the doctor-patient relationship. The earlier essay by Fred McMahon and Martin Zelder details the result: patients tend to overconsume health services; doctors, accountable to a state-set billing schedule and not to their patients, tend to oversupply health services; administrators protect turf.

By redefining insurance to mean zero payment, health care costs soar. Not surprisingly, then, provincial governments must work to temper patient demand. Largely, this has been done by restricting the supply of health care: reducing the number of medical graduates, running MRI scanners at bankers' hours, closing acute care beds, de-insuring services. Health care is rationed. It's like the old Soviet system where everything is free and nothing is readily available.

MSAs offer a way out of the quagmire. Instead of trying to reduce costs by reducing access to health care, MSAs reinvigorate the doctor-patient relationship with financial ties. Health care delivery thus becomes more efficient.

As we shall see in the following pages, MSAs are a popular idea in several countries. While the models differ — not simply among countries but even within them — MSAs are based on three very simple principles:

• Minor health expenses (what economists term "discretionary spending") are treated differently than major expenses (termed "catastrophic expenses").

- There is incentive for people to spend wisely.
- Insurance protects people against major expenses.

3. The United States

Canadians have a jaundiced — and a largely incorrect — view of American health care. Despite perceptions of a radical free market system, U.S. federal and state governments involve themselves in both the funding and regulation of health care. And, like Canada, people don't pay for their health care. Friedman explains: "[M]ost payments to physicians or hospitals or other caregivers for medical care are made not by the patient but by a third party — an insurance company or employer or governmental body."

This invites major problems. As Friedman observes, "No third party is involved when we shop at a supermarket. We pay the supermarket clerk directly. The same for gasoline for our cars, clothes for our back, and so on down the line. Why, by contrast, are most medical payments made by third parties?"[9]

Third party payment in the United States developed over decades, partly because of the tax code. And while the evolution of third party payment in the United States is different from the creation of government-run health care in Canada, the economic problem is similar: patients have no incentive to be cost conscious and as the potential to spend on health care increases, cost controls are put in place by bureaucrats (provincial officials in Canada and health maintenance organization [HMO] employees in the U.S.), often to the dissatisfaction of patients. In Canada, we ration through wait lists. In the United States, managed care attempts to limit what patients have access to.

Not surprisingly, many Americans resent the proliferation of HMOs and other types of managed care. As a reaction, some employers and individuals are looking to MSA-like medical coverage.

In the early 1990s, Golden Rule Insurance struggled, like many companies, with the rising cost of health care. Golden Rule provides health coverage for their employees. Rather than consider managed care, Golden Rule's management offered employees an alternative: they could opt for an MSA. In 1993, the majority of employees — some 80 percent — chose the MSA plan. Over the next half decade, the popularity of the program grew. Today the MSA plan is the choice of 98 percent of employees.

To ensure that a major illness wouldn't bankrupt an employee, Golden

Rule provides catastrophic insurance — a policy that covers all expenses above $2,000 a year. Thus, an employee hit by a bus or stricken with cancer won't have to sell his house to pay for the medical bills. For minor health expenses such as yearly physicals, X-rays, and prenatal care, the company deposits $1,000 in a special medical savings account, or MSA. When an employee needs minor medical attention, she simply pays for it from her MSA. For families, catastrophic coverage begins at $3,000, with $2,000 put into the MSA.

The popularity of the program isn't surprising. When an employee wants to see a doctor, there is no form to be filled out or permission to be granted from an HMO bureaucrat. The employee simply goes to the doctor and pays for the visit using the MSA. As an incentive for the employee to spend wisely, Golden Rule allows money remaining in the account at the end of the year to be withdrawn and spent freely. For the average employee, this translates into a handsome annual bonus.

MSAs also offer employees new choices. Since they have cash on hand to pay for health services, they can purchase preventive care. According to the vice-president's office, a full 20 percent of employees reported in 1994 that they purchased services they wouldn't have under traditional insurance. Today the number is closer to 26 percent.

And, for the management of Golden Rule, MSAs have meant a drop in health care costs. Major health expenses dropped in 1994 by 40 percent. This drop isn't surprising, as there is an incentive for patients to think before they use health services. Golden Rule Insurance has been so impressed with the approach that the company now offers this type of health insurance for other companies.

Other corporations, too, have embraced MSAs:

- *United Mine Workers Union.* Because of the appeal of MSAs, the union negotiated MSA-style health coverage for the 15,000 employees of Bituminous Coal Operators Association. Miners are provided with a high-deductible insurance and a $1,000 bonus at the start of each year to be used for health expenses.[10]

- *Quaker Oats.* The cereal manufacturer provides workers with a high-deductible insurance. The company also deposits $300 in an MSA. Over the first ten years of the plan, health costs grew by 6.3 percent annually. In the rest of the country, growth rates were more than 10 percent.[11]

- *Jersey City.* Employees of Jersey City, NJ can choose between traditional insurance and an MSA plan. In the latter, an insurance policy covers all expenses over $1,500 for individuals and $2,000 for families. The city then puts $1,500 and $2,000, respectively, in the MSA accounts of these employees. Workers can withdraw all unspent MSA money at the end of the year. Even though workers can withdraw up to $2,000 a year, the city finds that, because of reduced administrative costs, medical expenses are lower with the MSA plan.[12]

While MSA-based plans are still limited in number, the concept has gained favour in influential circles, including an endorsement from the American Medical Association.

The number of people actually covered by a tax-recognized MSA is only around 100,000 because of legislative restrictions. But many companies subscribe their employees to MSA-like plans (that is, plans that are conceptually similar to MSAs but don't meet the technical requirements of the relevant legislation to be formally called medical savings accounts).[13]

Destiny Health, the company mentioned at the beginning of this essay, offers just such a plan. Under a Destiny Health policy, an individual has complete coverage (i.e., no user fee or deductible) for any hospital stay, outpatient surgery, or chronic illness–related medication. For other health expenses (what Destiny Health terms "day-to-day benefits") individuals pay out of a "personal medical fund." Additional costs are first paid out-of-pocket and then out of a safety net. The financial incentive for day-to-day benefits is clear: at year's end, unspent money in the personal medical fund can be applied against the next year's potential out-of-pocket expenses or other health services.

The difference between Destiny Health's "personal medical fund" and a proper MSA is modest. Given Congress's reluctance to change legislation governing MSAs, it seems that relatively few will ever be covered by such insurance. But as fatigue grows with the restrictive nature of managed care, the general concept — as embodied in plans like the ones offered by Destiny Health — will surely become more popular.

Of course, there is a larger question: Is this a positive development?

Part and parcel of MSAs, of course, is the concept of providing individuals with a financial incentive *not* to spend money. For employees of Golden Rule, unspent monies can be withdrawn. In Singapore, Medisave monies accrue and can eventually be willed off or used for long-term care.

But do people really respond to these types of incentives? In a sense, part of the MSA system is the putting into place of some financial disincentive. Does this really reduce costs? How does this effect health outcomes?

In the 1970s, the California-based RAND think tank examined the impact of cost sharing on health expenses. It tapped the expertise of some of the top scholars in the world to design an experiment that would measure (1) the effects of price on consumption and (2) the health of those involved (health outcome). The RAND Health Insurance Experiment proved to be one of the largest and longest running social science research projects ever completed. Headed by Harvard Professor Joseph P. Newhouse, it involved approximately 2,000 nonelderly families and ran from 1974 to 1982. The cost was a staggering $136 million (U.S.$ in 1984).

The most interesting aspect of the experiment involved the use of medical services (additional work was done on dental and mental health services). Families were assigned two fundamentally different types of health insurance: a *free-care plan* and a *user-fee plan*. Those with the free-care plan paid no out-of-pocket expenses; visits to the family physician were free, as were visits to the emergency room. Those with the user-fee plan paid a certain percentage of cost up to a maximum of $1,000, depending on family income.

What did RAND find? "Use of medical services responds unequivocally to changes in the amount paid out of pocket."[14] It turns out that individual expenses in the free-care plan were 45 percent higher than those in the user-fee plan.

Comparing the free-care group with the user-fee group, RAND found that the free-care people were more likely to use medical services (28 percent more often), see a physician more regularly (67 percent more visits), and be admitted to a hospital (30 percent more frequently).

There's still the unresolved issue: What effect did user fees have on the health of individuals? The user-fee group used fewer medical services, but were the people in the group sicker as a result? Again the conclusion was unequivocal: "Our results show that the . . . increase in services had little or no measurable effect on health status for the average adult."[15] Those with the free-care plan used far more services, at far greater expense, without improving their overall health. In addition, there was no significant difference between the two groups in the risk of dying or in measures of pain and worry.[16]

4. South Africa and China

From a distance, South Africa and China have little in common. But in the early 1990s, both governments faced a similar woe: rising health costs. In

South Africa, the Mandela government attempted to reduce public expenses by encouraging more private insurance. For the Chinese, an attempt to find a solution rested with a government effort to control costs. Thus, experimentation in China focused on government measures while experimentation in South Africa took place largely in the private sector. But here's the surprise: despite their different approaches, MSAs are rapidly growing in both nations.

For most of the 1990s, South Africa had enjoyed one of the freest health insurance markets. Under President Nelson Mandela, regulations governing private insurance were greatly relaxed in 1994. As a result, South African insurance companies had flexibility to innovate and experiment (something much more difficult to achieve in a highly regulated market such as the one in the United States).

South Africans willing to pay for health insurance were thus allowed a large variety of insurance options, including numerous variants on American-style managed care plans (like HMOs).[17] Amazingly, within just five years, MSA-based plans became the most popular private insurance option, covering more than 4.6 million people.[18]

Different companies offer different policies, but a typical plan offers an individual an account of $685 with the catastrophic insurance kicking in at $1,100. But for many illnesses, there is no deductible for the catastrophic insurance. A patient requiring heart surgery, for instance, pays nothing out-of-pocket.

It's difficult not to marvel at the innovation of some plans. Discovery Health (the parent company of Destiny Health) introduced a wellness program called Vitality. Participants receive points for healthy decisions like joining a health club, or engaging in preventive health care (that is, getting regular Pap smears and mammograms). The points can be redeemed for a variety of prizes, including discounts on airline tickets. Discovery Health also offers patients a toll-free hotline, allowing them to speak with an experienced nurse day or night. Other companies have been creative, too. One policy offers a system for electronically verifying MSA balances and third party liability at the time prescription drugs are purchased.[19]

South African actuary Shaun Matisonn notes that MSA plans encourage people to cut their noncatastrophic expenses by more than half, on average.[20] "South Africa's experience with MSAs shows that MSA holders save money, spending less on discretionary items in a way that does not increase the cost of inpatient care. Contrary to allegations by some critics, the South African experience also shows that MSAs attract individuals of all different ages and different degrees of health."[21]

China introduced a variant of MSAs for citizens in two cities, Zhenjiang and Jiujiang.[22] Though the model is dictated by government officials — rather than an innovative private insurance market — the set up is recognizable. There are three levels of payment: a medical savings account, out-of-pocket spending, and a social risk pool (like a community-built catastrophic insurance).

Employees and employers contribute 1 percent and 10 percent, respectively, of their total wage bill each year. The 11 percent is divided between an individual account (6 percent) and a social risk pool (5 percent). When an individual uses a health service, payment comes out of the MSA. Any amount left over at the end of the year is rolled into the following year's account. When a MSA fund is exhausted, an individual must pay from his or her own pocket, up to 5 percent of annual income. Anything above this level is considered catastrophic and is largely paid from the community's social risk pool.

Although the experiment is still new, impressive results are already being realized. In one year, real health spending per beneficiary decreased by 27 percent. This result is all the more remarkable given that in neighbouring cities, where citizens still enjoy "free" health care, spending grew by 35 to 40 percent. Interestingly, savings weren't derived from fewer hospital stays or physician visits. The savings came from decreased use of diagnostic tests and expensive pharmaceuticals. The number of X-rays, for example, declined by more than half.

Impressed with these results, Chinese planners hope to extend the new health coverage to include 70 percent of the urban population.[23]

5. MSAs at Home: Some Questions and Answers

There are several experiments with MSAs outside of Canada, as outlined in this essay. Other jurisdictions are contemplating the implementation of this idea; recent news stories suggest great interest in both South Korea and Hong Kong. But are MSAs the sort of concept to consider here and how might they work? Let's answer some basic questions.

Why MSAs for Canada?

A colleague tells the story of how his home province solved the problem of waiting times for heart bypass surgery. "We don't have them here," he explained. How is it possible that his province, unlike any other in the country, doesn't have waiting times? "It's simple. We deal with everything on an emergency, ad hoc basis." No planning, the reasoning goes, no waiting times. My colleague wasn't joking, either. He relates the advice a cardiologist gives to some of his patients in that province: "Go to the emergency room and demand the surgery. And don't leave until you get it."

These stories are typical in Canada. We wait for practically any diagnostic test, procedure, or surgery.

But the root cause of this problem isn't a lack of funding or lack of administrative reform. We have never spent more on health care than we do today (and, internationally, we rank third in total spending as a percentage of the GDP). We have never attempted to micromanage this system more than we do now.

Rather, we are seeing the end result of medicare's structural flaw. By making all health care free, the doctor-patient relationship has been corrupted. As noted earlier in this essay, patients tend to overconsume health resources and doctors tend to overprovide services. Health reforms for the past thirty years have attempted to address this problem. But a structural flaw cannot be outregulated or micromanaged away.

MSAs would reinvigorate the doctor-patient relationship with financial ties. This approach is in stark contrast with the present "reforms": instead of more government planning, we would look to a system built on individual choice and competition.

Various models of MSAs have different degrees of government involvement. But even in the most libertarian approach, MSAs still require a major role for government to play: to provide for the poor and chronically ill and to regulate. But this is an appropriate role for the government to take. Consider that with food, the state provides welfare so that those who cannot afford bread or meat can purchase it. The government does not, however, nationalize food production and distribution and then set up regional food boards to determine how many slices of salami a neighbourhood needs.

How Would MSAs Work?

Because any change to medicare is deemed "right-wing," people automatically assume that the concept of MSAs must involve private insurance companies and private hospitals.

There are good reasons to favour an increased role for private medicine, both in an unreformed medicare system and an MSA-based health care system, but MSAs themselves are ideologically neutral. If all private involvement in health care is deemed a bad idea — a view often proposed by medicare's most ardent supporters — it would still be possible to have a government-run and government-financed MSA system. Socialism is not incompatible with MSAs, as illustrated by the Chinese experiment.

The basic principle is this: Individual choice and competition is better than bureaucratic management. To this end, small expenses are paid out of an account, with a financial incentive in place to ensure that people are frugal; major expenses are covered by insurance.

But who would fund these accounts? There are three basic financing models:

- In the government model, each Canadian would be allocated a certain amount of money every year for his or her health expenses. Demographics, gender, health status, and geographic base would determine the amount. People would be required to get catastrophic insurance, again provided by the government.
- In the private model, Canadians would allocate a certain percentage of their income to a tax-free MSA account. Catastrophic insurance would be required, but would be purchased from private (and regulated) insurance companies.
- In the mixed model there would be something in between, such as public funding of the accounts with the option to buy private catastrophic insurance.

The level of private involvement would also depend on the model. In China, government insurance pays for public system doctors and public system hospitals. In South Africa, MSA holders pick from private doctors and private hospitals. Singapore's system offers a mix, with public and private hospitals competing for business.

No matter how public or private the MSA system, the three principles outlined earlier — minor health expenses are treated differently than major expenses; there is incentive for people to spend wisely; insurance protects people against major expenses — would need to be satisfied.

Are MSAs Just Glorified User Fees?

Part of the attraction of MSAs is the fact that individuals have an incentive to think twice before accessing services for lesser health expenses.

That's no small matter. When people think about health care, they imagine emergency care: dreadful car accidents, complicated surgeries, and other exciting events that make *ER* a popular television show. Obviously, there isn't much of a decision to make about, say, going to an emergency room after a major motor vehicle accident.

But most of health care does not, in fact, involve spectacular life-saving measures. You can visualize health care spending as a triangle, in which each contact with medicine is represented by a point in that triangle. The distance of the point from the base represents the cost of care. Most points are close to the base: trips to the doctor for a physical exam or an eye infection, the occasional ankle sprain, healthy baby check-ups. Higher up the triangle, care becomes more expensive (and more rare): in-patient hospital stays, surgeries, extensive rehabilitation. At the apex, there are highly expensive procedures, such as transplants. Few people ever experience care at the apex.

In order to reduce cost, we presently ration through waiting. There are long delays for getting diagnostic tests or specialist consults. By encouraging patients to be more accountable for their decisions, this type of rationing would be unnecessary.

But MSAs are more than glorified user fees. MSAs would introduce a competitive health care environment. Presently, patients use the health care system. With MSAs, they would become customers of the health care system.

As in Singapore, the result would be lower-cost, higher-quality care. (Actually, in Canada, competition can be observed in the private MRI market. Scans used to cost more than $800 in Edmonton. Today, it is possible to get this diagnostic test done for hundreds less.) As opposed to worrying about the protection of turf, administrators would start competing for patient dollars. An MSA dollar goes to the user, who chooses how to spend it. If a hospital has many administrators and high overhead costs, its services will cost more. Patients then will be tempted to go to a better-run and lower-cost hospital. A more efficient system would be the result.

The most immediate result would be the end of waiting lists. If waiting lists develop within an MSA system, they won't be tolerated (and certainly not encouraged) but, rather, viewed as a bottleneck. Because health care providers under such a system compete for patient funding, the bottleneck will be viewed as an opportunity — providers will have a direct financial incentive to address the problem, whether by hiring more nurses and technicians or by acquiring new equipment and facilities. Remember that in Canada, shortages rarely occur with, say, food. At Christmas time, when consumers demand more fruitcake, bakers respond — they have a financial interest to do so. The problem with the health care system today is that no one really has a financial interest.

And providers would innovate. Imagine clinics that emphasize preventive care, twenty-four-hour call services, and other services that get flouted in public policy circles today. The same innovative forces that have replaced the dreary cup of coffee with latte and have slashed the hourly rate of Internet services would be applied to health care.

What about the Aging of the Population?

One the biggest challenges facing Canada's health care system is the aging of our population. In his essay on demographics earlier in this volume, David Baxter notes the coming crunch. If the system is stretched today, what will it look like in the future?

MSAs can us help deal with the aging issue. First, MSAs would make the present system more efficient. As opposed to an unregulated government monopoly, our health care system would be patient-centred and competitive. This would save money.

Second, since many people would have unspent money in their MSAs, it would be easy to see this arrangement evolving into a type of RRSP-system for health care. Unspent monies could be invested, allowing interest to accrue.

Wouldn't People Neglect Their Health?

The strongest argument against MSAs is that provided with an incentive to be frugal, people would be too hesitant to see their doctor. Would a person who religiously clips coupons and buys yogurt by the flat to save money be the best judge of his or her health care needs?

As discussed earlier, the California think tank RAND tracked 2,000 families over eight years in a study that cost more than U.S.$100 million in 1984. The study compared the health and the health care spending of two groups: one with free health care and the other with user fees for services. The result? People on the free-care plan spent significantly more but in the end were no healthier than those on the user-fee plan. The lack of difference in overall health status between the two groups proves that patients are able to make intelligent health care choices when provided with the financial incentive to do so.

There's a further argument in favour of MSAs: they may actually make people healthier than the present system. Because account holders would have cash on hand, they could utilize more preventive health care than they currently do. The experience of Golden Rule employees supports this argument: a quarter of the people with MSAs reported that they used preventive care they previously hadn't. A two-year, random trial involving 43,000 employees of Dupont found that sick days were reduced by 14 percent through a health education initiative. Such a result isn't isolated. In a recent article in *Health Affairs*, former U.S. Surgeon General C. Everett Koop and four coauthors reviewed thirty-two programs and found that such efforts generally reduced health insurance claims by 20 percent.[24]

The present health care system doesn't do much to encourage preventive care. By making money for such services readily available and by increasing people's consciousness of health care costs, MSAs could change current attitudes.

What about the Poor and the Chronically Ill?

The government will need to provide for these two groups.

Of course, this need is dependent on the way MSAs are financed. If the government gives every citizen and/or family a certain amount of money for their MSA, the poor — like the middle class and the affluent — would receive the same grant. Alternatively, if MSA funding were done privately, then the government would need to give a special grant to the poor and the chronically ill, as is done in Singapore. The government may also fill the gap between the MSA and the catastrophic insurance for the poor.

NOTES

1. Thomas A. Massaro and Yu-Ning Wong, "Medical Savings Accounts: The Singapore Experience," *NCPA Report No. 203*, Apr. 1996, 2.
2. Lee Kuan Yew, *From Third World To First: The Singapore Story: 1965–2000* (New York: HarperCollins Publishing, 2000), 96.

3. Ibid., 100–02.
4. The following figures are based on Kai Hong Phua, "Medical Savings Accounts and Health Care Financing in Singapore," World Bank discussion paper No. 365, Innovations in Health Care Financing: Proceedings of a World Bank Conference, Washington DC, 10–11 Mar. 1997.
5. Tricia Edmonds, personal correspondence with author, 6 Sept. 2001.
6. Cynthia Ramsay, personal correspondence with author, 1 Oct. 2001.
7. Thomas Massaro, personal correspondence with author, 5 Mar. 2001.
8. Milton Friedman, "How to Cure Health Care," *The Public Interest*, Winter 2001, www.thepublicinterest.com/archives/2001/winter/article1.html.
9. Ibid.
10. Peter J. Ferrara, "More than a Theory: Medical Savings Accounts at Work," Cato Institute, Washington, DC, Policy Analysis 220, 14 Mar. 1995, 15–16.
11. Ibid., 14.
12. Ibid., 15.
13. The more general category of "defined contributions" — where employers give their employees money to spend on health care — covers roughly 10 percent of the private insurance market.
14. Joseph P. Newhouse and the Insurance Experiment Group, *Free for All? Lessons from the RAND Health Insurance Experiment* (Cambridge: Harvard University Press, 1993), 40.
15. Ibid., 243.
16. The RAND researchers noted that in only one instance did the free-care plan have an advantage over the user-fee plan: for poor people with high blood pressure. The authors conclude, however, that "a one-time screening examination achieved most of the gain in blood pressure that free care achieved."
17. Laura B. Benko, "High Interest Rate: South Africa's Experience with MSAs is Worlds Apart from America's," *Modern Healthcare International*, 13 Nov. 2000, 38.
18. Ibid.
19. Shaun Matisonn, "Medical Savings Accounts in South Africa," NCPA *Policy Report No. 234*, June 2000, 2.
20. For younger families, MSAs reduced expenses by 56 percent. Households headed by seniors enjoyed a 47 percent reduction. Inpatient costs fell by 81 percent for younger families and 73 percent for older ones.
21. Matisonn, "Medical Savings Accounts," 20.
22. William C. Hsiao, Winnie C. Yip, and Chevy Chase, "Medical Savings Accounts: Lessons from China," *Health Affairs*, Nov./Dec. 1997, 244–51.
23. Jeremy Page, "Chinese move toward private health insurance," Reuters, 18 Jan. 2000.
24. C. Everett Koop et al., "Beyond Health Promotion: Reducing the Need and Demand for Medical Care," *Health Affairs* 17.2 (1998): 70–84.

FINAL THOUGHTS

Will it ever change?

That's the most common question I'm asked. Whether it's at a meeting of administrators, in a radio interview, or at a casual gathering of friends, someone eventually will pop the big question.

People wonder if our health care system will ever really change. Certainly, there are many reasons to argue that it won't. Politicians are fearful of this issue. Special interests are aggressive and well organized. The public is divided. If no one is ready to champion reform, how can real change ever take place?

Not that long ago, my favourite journalist reminded me of Stein's Law. Economist Herbert Stein led an exceptional life: he chaired the President's Council of Economic Advisers, penned several books, and wrote frequently for the *Wall Street Journal*. Perhaps Stein's most memorable contribution, however, was a simple observation: That which cannot go on forever will eventually stop.

Will health care ever change? We already know the answer. Our health care system is under incredible stress. ERs routinely overcrowd. Waiting lists exist for practically every procedure and diagnostic test. Patients suffer. Far from being resolved in the near future, the problems with Canadian health care will worsen with time. The population is aging — a burden in and of itself — just as the "high-tech, high-expense" medical revolution is transforming care. The proper question to ask is not "Will medicare change?" but "When will medicare change?" Do we embark upon the path to reform now or wait until the system collapses from inertia and neglect?

Sadly, some see public policy through the prism of national identity. They will oppose any significant change to the system. At a time when

Blairites in Britain are entertaining the concept of privatization and central planners in China are recognizing the need for patient cost sharing, they are adamant that we must embrace the sinking status quo. They wrap themselves in the Canadian flag, but is that acceptable? Is allowing cancer patients to wait months for treatment the mark of citizenship? Is allowing our elderly to lie on stretchers in hospital ERs for days the best way to be un-American? Beware the cruel reality of well-intentioned nationalism.

There are no easy changes to make. There is, however, a path worth pursuing. Rather than increasing bureaucratic control or blindly throwing more money at medicare, we should look to reforming health care along the lines of individual choice and competition. Internationally, there are practices worth considering: public-private partnerships, user fees, private insurance. Any step toward reform ought to begin with some experimentation with these initiatives. We should go further, too, and try medical savings accounts.

Much has been written about the 1960s and 1970s. If the reformers of those two decades suffered failures, they also achieved great changes. It was during those years that civil rights, for example, were accepted. Those years also saw federal and provincial politicians get together to address the problems with medical care. Looking back on that period, we see people who dreamed of a better world and fought for the innovation and change necessary to make it possible.

We must dream again. Our task is daunting. But remember, there is only one alternative and Stein's Law predicts the long-term result. Canadians deserve better.

NOTES ON CONTRIBUTORS

David Baxter, a Vancouver-based demographer, is the executive director of The Urban Futures Institute. An author of reports, papers, and textbooks, Baxter writes on numerous topics, from market trends to population growth. He is a popular conference speaker and addresses more than fifty organizations every year. He has held professorships at the University of British Columbia and the Asian Institute of Technology, and is often quoted in newspapers such as the *Globe and Mail*, *National Post*, and *Vancouver Sun*.

Michael Bliss is a professor of history and the history of medicine at the University of Toronto. He is the author of ten books, including *The Discovery of Insulin*, *Right Honourable Men*, and *William Osler: A Life in Medicine*. Bliss's work has received numerous honours, ranging from the Sir John A. Macdonald Prize of the Canadian Historical Association to a National Business Book Award. He has been appointed a member of the Order of Canada and elected a fellow of the Royal Society of Canada. Professor Bliss also writes for a variety of popular publications, including the *National Post* and *Time*.

J. Edwin Coffey is a retired physician, a specialist in gynecology and obstetrics. He trained at the Johns Hopkins Hospital in Baltimore. In Montreal he practised at both the Montreal General and Royal Victoria hospitals and was an associate professor at McGill's Faculty of Medicine. He is a former president of the Quebec Medical Association and has served on the Board of the Canadian Medical Association and its Working Group on Health Care Financing in Canada. He is currently a research associate at the Montreal Economic Institute where he writes on health reform.

Brian Lee Crowley is the founding president of the Atlantic Institute for Market Studies. Crowley writes extensively on public policy issues and is a former member of the editorial board at the *Globe and Mail*. Crowley has held a variety of positions, both in and out of academia, including president of the Atlantic Provinces Economic Council, government advisor on constitutional and electoral reform issues, diplomat for the EEC Commission, aid administrator for the UN in Africa, and professor at Dalhousie University. He holds a doctorate in political economy from the London School of Economics. With David Zitner, Crowley is coauthor of *Operating in the Dark*, winner of the prestigious Sir Anthony Fisher Award.

David R. Henderson is a research fellow at Stanford University's Hoover Institution and an economics professor at the Naval Postgraduate School in Monterey, CA. He has contributed numerous articles to *Fortune*, the *Wall Street Journal*, and the *Chicago Tribune*. Henderson is the editor of *The Fortune Encyclopedia of Economics* (translated into two other languages) and recently wrote *The Joy of Freedom: An Economist's Odessey*. He served as the senior health economist with the President's Council of Economic Advisers (1982–84). A Canadian by birth, he earned his Bachelor of Science degree from the University of Winnipeg.

Johan Hjertqvist advises the Greater Stockholm Council in Sweden on health care policy. He has successively been an entrepreneur, a consultant, and a deputy mayor of the Swedish city of Tyreso. He writes extensively on the reform of social services and has published books on the topic. He is a research director with Timbro, a Swedish think tank, and oversees "Health in Transition," a four-year pilot project whose objective is to describe and analyze the operation of a competitive market within the public health system.

Carl Irvine is a Toronto-based economist. He is presently a doctoral candidate at the University of Toronto (economics) where his academic work focuses on public policy issues such as taxation and health care. Irvine is coauthor of a paper with economist Martin Zelder on private health insurance and the uninsured in the United States (forthcoming from the Fraser Institute). He has also written on American Medicaid and regulatory changes in the late 1980s.

Fred McMahon is the director of the Social Affairs Centre at the Fraser Institute. He is the author of three books, as well as numerous articles and papers. *Looking the Gift Horse in the Mouth: The Impact of Federal Transfers on Atlantic Canada* won the Sir Anthony Fisher International Memorial Award for advancing public policy debate. *Retreat from Growth: Atlantic Canada and the Negative Sum Economy* was shortlisted for the 2000 Donner Prize for best book on public policy. He has worked for the Consumer Policy Institute, the Atlantic Institute for Market Studies, and the Bank of Canada.

William Orovan is a surgeon, specializing in urology. He is a professor at McMaster University and is chair of the Department of Surgery. Orovan's diverse career includes work as a business consultant. He has also held a variety of administrative positions: chief of the department of surgery and chief of medical staff at St. Joseph's Hospital (twelve years and four years, respectively), board member of the Ontario Medical Association (eight years) and chief negotiator (six years), and interim dean of McMaster's Faculty of Health Sciences. He has also served as the president of the OMA.

Cynthia Ramsay is a Vancouver-based health economist and consultant. She has worked at both Statistics Canada and the Fraser Institute. She has written more than 100 articles, briefs, and papers on health care, including the Fraser Institute's annual waiting list survey and a paper on medical savings accounts. Ramsay is coeditor of *Healthy Incentives: Canadian Health Reform in an International Context*, a collection of essays looking at health care in Canada and Europe. She is now publisher of the *Jewish Western Bulletin*.

Neil Seeman holds a Master's degree in public health (Harvard) and a Bachelor of Laws degree (University of Toronto). He is currently the senior researcher and in-house counsel for the National Citizens Coalition. Seeman also writes extensively about health care and politics, and has been published in newspapers on both sides of the border. He served on the editorial board of the *National Post* (1998–2001) and as an associate editor of the *National Review Online* (2001). He is an executive member of the Canadian Business and Economic Roundtable on Mental Health.

314 ◆ BETTER MEDICINE

William Watson is an economist who earned his doctorate at Yale University. He has taught at McGill University since 1977. He is best known for his newspaper columns on economics and other matters. He appears twice weekly in the *National Post* and edits the journal *Policy Options*. In 1997–98, he oversaw the editorial section of the *Ottawa Citizen*. His 1998 book, *Globalization and the Meaning of Canadian Life*, was runner-up for the Donner Prize for best public policy book. In 1989, he won a National Magazine Award gold medal in the humour category for a piece he published in *Saturday Night*.

Margaret Wente is a columnist for the *Globe and Mail* and writes about health care, education, and the way we currently live. Wente's career in journalism is diverse. She has edited two leading business magazines and helped launch the CBC Television show *Venture*. At the *Globe* she edited *Report on Business*, then served as managing editor in charge of daily news operations. During most of that time she also wrote a weekly column and, since 1999, she has been writing full time. Wente's work has won many awards over the years, including National Magazine Awards for both writing and editing and the National Newspaper Award for her *Globe* column.

Martin Zelder is an economist. He holds a doctorate from the University of Chicago, where his dissertation was supervised by Nobel laureate Gary S. Becker. He served as director of Health Policy Research at The Fraser Institute for several years and has held faculty positions at the College of William and Mary, The Australian National University, and Northwestern University. He is the author of several papers on Canadian health care that explore technology, funding, and waiting lists, and he has published articles in numerous newspapers.

David Zitner, a family doctor, is the director of Medical Informatics at the Dalhousie Medical School. He has served as a member of the Physician Advisory Committee for the Canadian Institute for Health Information and participated in the Federal/Provincial/Territorial Deputy Ministers of Health Working Group, which produced "When Less is Better: Using Canada's Hospitals Efficiently." He chairs the Utilization Committee for the QEII Health Sciences Centre in Halifax and is a member of the board for both the Nova Scotia Medical Society and the Canadian Council for Health Services Accreditation. With Brian Lee Crowley, Zitner is coauthor of *Operating in the Dark*, winner of the prestigious Sir Anthony Fisher Award.

INDEX